FEEL GOOD FOR MENOPAUSE

BY

AMANDA RYDER

Published by Well Women Publishing

Copyright © 2023 Amanda Ryder

ISBN: 978-1-3999-5425-9

Images by Leti Ryder

Book Cover Design by ebooklaunch.com

To the women in my life, past and present
– I'd be nothing without you

CONTENTS

in a position to make a positive contribution, helping women become the healthiest possible versions of themselves.

Now, back to menopause, and how perimenopause (the time around menopause when your hormones are declining but in an erratic fashion, a bit like puberty in reverse) affected me.

My perimenopause started in my mid-40s. Up until then, I'd always considered myself to be optimistic, energised and robust, the sort of person who would get up and go after what she wanted. I had embraced living in Spain for a decade, had felt resilient in terms of the ups and downs of life, had loved bringing up my kids, had loved my work and spending time with friends... generally, I was a happy camper. I'd also dedicated time to my fitness and nutrition, naively believing this made me bulletproof when it came to my menopause. Not so! I was totally unprepared for the array of (what I thought were) unrelated symptoms that ended up completely knocking me for six. Looking back at that time in my mid-40s, I can't believe how different I became – I'd lost sight of who I was, my confidence had waned, and I was merely a shadow of my former self. Horrible!

I wonder if you too can relate to this – do you feel like you're living a suboptimal life, settling for an existence you don't like, and feeling not at all like yourself? If you're not careful, menopause can really chip away at your identity, your positivity, and your can-do attitude.

Since that time in my mid-40s, I've focused on getting myself sorted, and now I spend my time helping women who find themselves in a similar situation. For many of us, this can be a challenging and isolating time. There are so many women struggling through every day, not understanding what's going on with their bodies and minds, and wondering why they feel so different all of a sudden. Sadly, most of these women believe they have no other option than to simply tough it out and settle for a 'new normal'.

My perimenopause kicked in at 46, at which point I started to feel insecure and anxious. I'd never suffered from anxiety before, so it was strange to say the least. I noticed that my thoughts were becoming quite dark, and that my glass-half-full attitude had completely disappeared! I also noticed that I had little to no tolerance for stress, that I became easily overwhelmed, and that even the slightest negative thought or musing (which were now coming thick and fast) would be enough to bring on a surge of heat that swept over me like a freak wave. My motivation and confidence levels were low to non-existent, and I was relying on wine and chocolate to cheer me up – letting go of some of my healthier, entrenched habits at the same time.

It left me completely perplexed, wondering what the hell had happened to me. I seemed so far from myself at that time – which was incredibly isolating in itself – and, on top of that, I felt ashamed and weak for feeling this way.

I'm not telling you this because I want sympathy – I'm fine now, don't worry! – but to demonstrate that there's no shame in talking about your menopausal experience and, therefore, normalising these common symptoms and experiences. After all, even the most robust woman can be knocked for six!

I hear so many similar stories from so many women who feel like they're no longer themselves, either physically or mentally. If, therefore, you've suddenly started feeling different or have noticed that menopausal symptoms have crept up on you over time, just remember: you're not alone. Really, it's no wonder we experience these changes so profoundly considering the hormonal equilibrium we've become accustomed to on every level for three decades suddenly shifts!

Of course, every woman's experience of menopause is different. For me, it was changes to my mood and anxiety levels, plus a few other physical issues. For you, it might be energy, weight gain, irritability, angry outbursts, sleep issues, hot flushes, and so on – the list is a long one. However, I want you to know that whatever afflictions you're experiencing, they can be helped or resolved if you know where to look. It's also possible to turn things around and feel much more like your old self again – and, in some ways, even better. I've worked with hundreds of women, helping them navigate their way through menopause, so that they too can tap into the joyful enthusiasm for life that our daughters, nieces, and all the young women around us seem to have in abundance. Who doesn't want to hang on to that *joie de vivre* for as long as they can?

I've written this book to share with you what I've learnt, as a woman and a clinician, to help you navigate this tricky time – because I fully appreciate just how challenging and stressful it can be when you feel you must accept a new way of being that isn't aligned with who you feel you really are.

I've seen how possible it is for my clients and friends to reconnect with the person they most identify with: their former selves. I would encourage you, therefore, not to settle for anything less.

Of course, it's also important to embrace this new era in your life, because I don't think it's a case of trying to stay young forever – personally, I hate the term 'anti-ageing' and prefer to think that we're all ageing with health and grace. Even though we can't escape time and the fact that we're growing older, it's preferable to embrace this new stage in our lives with dignity and with our heads held high. I believe, with the right attitude and the right techniques to help us keep on top of our health, we can halt all the worrying about ageing and time marching on. Instead, we can give ourselves freedom from time – because we're comfortable and confident with who we are, and the lives we wish to lead.

This is your recipe for thriving at menopause, midlife, or whatever you wish to call it.

INTRODUCTION

Menopause Really Chooses Its Moment!

If you're like a lot of women in their 40s and 50s, then you may have more on your plate than your younger self did. You may be taking care of ageing parents or teenage children, have a demanding job, be working long hours, and/or be at the height of your career, all while sleeping less and doing more. Perhaps you're still figuring out exactly what gives you purpose in life and how to live with all the uncertainty this inevitably brings up. It's no wonder that some of us women feel tired and emotional when all that resilience, energy, optimism, and motivation we had in previous decades just... recedes, right when we need it the most.

Throw all the fluctuating, declining hormones into the mix and you have the perfect storm!

It's Not All Doom And Gloom – The Truth Serum

However, I find that when I bring midlife women together, some talk about 'the truth serum' – the sudden ability to speak their minds and to stop compromising with themselves. Some say that, once they've got on top of their menopausal symptoms and have taken back control of their minds and bodies, they feel more fired up, more ambitious, and more open to new challenges.

Let's not be drawn into the narrative that menopause equals washed up, tired, irrelevant, unwell, and that your best years are behind you – which is what you're presented with if you google photos of a menopausal woman. I mean, come on... who of us really identifies with the image of a desperately sad-looking woman sitting in front of a fan trying to cool down during a hot flush?!

Instead, let's look to the women who are still rocking it in their 40s, 50s, and 60s, and find inspiration from them. Women like Emma Walmsley (CEO of GSK), Deborah Meaden, Kristin Scott Thomas, Gabby Logan, Michelle Obama, Susannah Reid, and Kate Bingham (who led the government vaccine strategy), just to mention a few! These women are creative, bold, courageous, hard-working, authentic, and happy in their own skins – even after midlife.

I'm not saying we should all be chasing a big job or a TV career; what I'm saying is that we all deserve the energy, freedom, and motivation we need to live the life that's true to who we are. Whether it's continuing your work, exploring your creative side, or getting the most out of being with your family and friends, we shouldn't have to give into the feeling that we're somehow compromised, more vulnerable, less relevant, or that we lack the confidence to do what we want with our lives, especially when we reflect on all the life experience we have under our belts.

What About Us?

Over the years, I've noticed that I'm far more able to handle stress and life's challenges when I'm feeling happy, relaxed, and energised – and I'm sure this is true for most of us. These feelings, however, can be sadly lacking at midlife. Without the energy, motivation, and *joie de vivre* we usually have, it's impossible to pursue our interests, work on our careers, do regular exercise, eat well, and generally take care of ourselves and those around us. What kind of life is that?

So, let's get started, so you can start to feel better! If you're one of the lucky ones with no symptoms, however, it's still important to understand the effects that lower hormone levels can have on our bodies – especially our bones, brain, and heart health. We need to pay more attention to our health right now, because – even if you don't notice any changes – your body is currently shifting and adjusting to a new normal.

There's no getting away from it: menopause changes us. And that robust body of yours, which used to get away with overindulging, rushing around, late nights, too much alcohol, gruelling workouts, and handling stress, is no longer able to cope with those same demands. However, once you put a set of healthy habits in place, you'll discover something wonderful: your resilience can be restored.

More Than Good Advice

"He who has a why can bear almost any how" – Viktor Frankl.

What most of us need to understand – when we're embracing change and taking on new advice – is the **why**, as well as the motivation and inspiration needed to pick up new, sustainable habits. It's one thing knowing what you're supposed to do, but quite another to actually do it. My aim is to give you the practical guidance you need in all areas of your life.

I'll share my expertise on nutrition and lifestyle, plus my take on hormone replacement therapy, as well as imparting what I've learnt from working with women – including what really gets results! Most of the book is dedicated to helping you instil healthy habits you can live by, such as 'the feel-good four' (essential in putting a satisfying meal together) and 'legumes for lunch', as well as how to incorporate helpful phytoestrogens into your diet. There's also advice on how you can avoid weight gain – and how to lose some weight, if necessary.

The objective here is to ensure you're fully informed so that you can make the best choices for you as an individual. Why not give yourself every advantage so that you're more likely to age gracefully with energy, optimism, and good health? Going forward, I really hope I can inspire and motivate you to be the best, happiest version of yourself.

So, before we delve in, I'd first like to give you an explanation of what is happening to your body throughout your 40s and 50s – and beyond – so you can fully understand this natural process and why it has such an impact on you.

It's worth bearing in mind that, all being well, we're going to spend a third of our life post-menopause, so it's vital we get it right. After all, most of us are incredibly experienced by this point in our lives, having banked a lot of life skills and wisdom – and we still have so much more to contribute. I have a friend who says: 'Each time I complain about being 50, I remind myself of the alternative.' Certainly food for thought.

Who Knew?

Did you know that we are one of the few mammals who actually live past our reproductive years? Yes, it's just us and a handful of whales – orcas being one. Most go on having offspring right up to the end – and I'm not sure I like the sound of that!

CHAPTER 1 ~ FEEL GOOD ABOUT THE CHANGES

Why Men And Women Experience Midlife Differently

Women's hormones tend to decline more quickly than men's, hence we feel the symptoms of midlife more abruptly and therefore have a lot more to deal with!

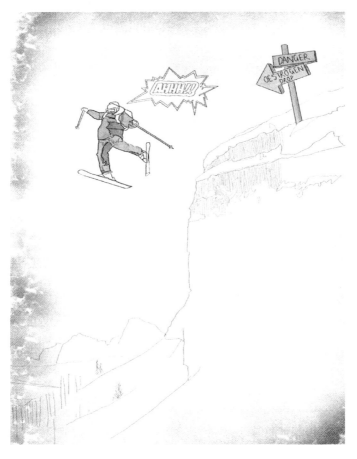

Danger: Oestrogen Drop!

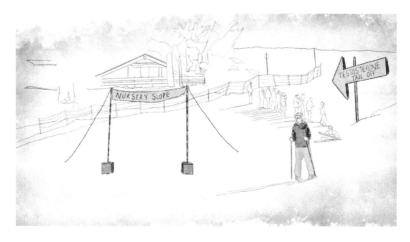

Men's hormones, on the other hand, decline in a slow, steady fashion over many years, hence why they don't feel the consequences as suddenly.

It's as if, one day, you're feeling fine – and musing that menopause must just be something that happens to other women, best not to think about it, right? – and then, suddenly, YOU start to experience some surprising symptoms... and you may only be in your 40s!

You may have regular periods at this point, or you may find you have a cycle every two weeks for a couple of cycles and then nothing for a few months. Other women find that their period is just lost in action, never to return, whilst some find their periods are much heavier, more troublesome, and more frequent than before. Everyone's transition is different.

Some women find that they start getting warmer, experiencing night sweats, and waking up more at night – especially after too much stress, coffee, or alcohol, as they're unable to tolerate these like they used to. Some find that they've lost their libido, or that they're feeling anxious; one friend joked that she'd wake up in the middle of the night, realise she'd forgotten to send a birthday card to a distant cousin, and that would be enough to trigger an anxiety attack, insomnia, and a hot flush!

It's easy to see how your normal life – with its usual trials and tribulations – can suddenly become rather overwhelming.

Have You Fallen Off The Happy Train?

We may also experience a low mood, low self-esteem, and depression, as well as gaining weight – especially around the middle! We may find ourselves yo-yoing between happiness and the depths of despair, feeling irritable, angry, and tired, or we may experience headaches, migraines, a lack of confidence, brain fog, feeling more achy than usual… the list goes on and on (just google the 34 symptoms of menopause for a comprehensive list – there's everything from dry eyes to burning tongue syndrome). You may experience one of these symptoms or all of them – we're all different – and, to add to the confusion, these symptoms will come and go, so you often start doubting yourself and your symptoms!

So, where are you in terms of your menopause? There are three stages:

Perimenopause

This simply means the transition from having periods until they stop – and this can start up to 5-10 years before your period stops altogether. It's a bit of a roller coaster, with several highs and lows.

Menopause (meno – month, pause – to cease)

This is when you haven't had a period for 12 consecutive months, and it comes just before postmenopause. So, in reality, menopause really only lasts for one day: the day you reach 12 months without a period. This happens at an average age of 51.

Hence, we spend more time being perimenopausal and post-menopausal than menopausal.

Postmenopause

The time after your menopause.

(Please note: in this book I'll often just use the word menopause to cover both perimenopause and postmenopause.)

In the pink / changing oestrogen levels over a women's lifetime

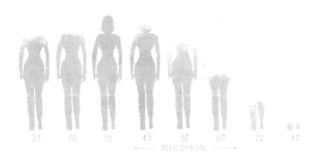

The symptoms we experience occur because, around this time, our ovaries start to significantly reduce the amount of oestrogen and progesterone they secrete due to a lack of viable eggs. The transition to menopause can certainly be a bumpy ride as our hormones decline. However, this is usually done in a fluctuating fashion, as they rise and fall erratically on their way down. This is known as the perimenopause or the time around menopause.

> **What Are Hormones?** Hormones are chemicals that are made from the glands in our bodies. Essentially, they are messengers that tell parts of our body how and when to work. They control development and growth, metabolism of food, sexual function, fertility, brain function, mood, and body temperature. When they're out of balance, we really know about it!

When it comes to hormones, which are powerful chemical messengers in the body, a little goes a long way – we feel their effects deeply. Oestrogen receptor sites are found all over the body, not just in our reproductive organs: they're in our brain, immune cells, bones, joints, muscles, gastrointestinal tract, uterus, ovaries, cardiovascular system, skin, breasts, bladder, vagina, eyes, heart, lungs, blood vessels... literally everywhere! It's really no wonder we feel oestrogen's absence so acutely.

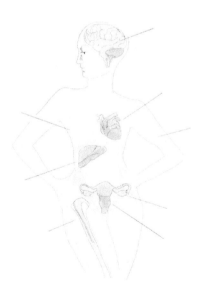

The good news is, once you get on top of any symptoms and have made your way through the transition, you may find there's a lot to celebrate: no more periods, no more PMT, more headspace, the ability to speak your mind, and more focus on your passion/career.

If you can't speak your mind now, when can you? Go for it!

When It Comes To Hormones, Balance Is A Key Factor

Whilst we don't have that much control over our sex hormones (oestrogen, progesterone, and testosterone), we can influence two very important hormones: **insulin** and **cortisol**. Throughout this book, I will explain how you can positively influence these two hormones, which will have a major impact on your health and wellbeing.

Adios, Progesterone

Usually, the first hormone to drop off is progesterone – this is because, during our perimenopause, we ovulate less often. The corpus luteum, which is just the shell left over once we've ovulated, is responsible for producing progesterone. So, no ovulation equals no progesterone.

Progesterone can help us feel calm, reduce anxiety, and promote a good night's sleep. For some women, therefore, one of the first symptoms they notice as they go through perimenopause is anxiety.

Oestrogen needs its calming sister, progesterone, to bring balance to the body. Therefore, if we produce less progesterone, our ratio of oestrogen to progesterone changes and we may start to experience anxiety. We may also notice other things like sleep disturbances, heavier periods, breast tenderness, headaches, and mood swings.

As perimenopause progresses and our lifetime supply of viable eggs declines, we are no longer able to produce oestrogen in the quantities our bodies are accustomed to, and that's when we really start to notice the change.

A little-known fact is that we make four times the amount of testosterone as we do oestrogen, so we can also feel the effects of low testosterone too. Low testosterone can affect our libido, motivation, energy, and confidence.

Each ovary is the size of a grape – so it's amazing how they can store up to 300-400,000 eggs by the time we reach puberty. Plus, throughout our reproductive years, we produce approximately 500 viable eggs – they're such busy little organs!

Once our ovaries have run out of eggs and shut up shop, we're no longer able to make these hormones in the quantities our bodies are used to. At this point, we're banking on our fat cells and our adrenal glands (the same glands that pump out the cortisol hormone) to take up the slack and make us some oestrogen. The health of our adrenal glands, therefore, is of paramount importance when it comes to our hormonal balance; stress can negatively impact the adrenal glands, reducing their ability to produce sufficient backup hormones. More on this later.

Are You Struggling With Weight Gain?

Many of us gain weight in midlife even when we're eating the same amount of food; this is because, as our oestrogen levels decline, we become less sensitive to the effects of insulin. This, in turn, can lead to a level of insulin resistance, resulting in worsening menopausal symptoms and weight gain. Insulin is the hormone responsible for removing glucose from the bloodstream and placing it in our cells. It is also a fat-storage hormone; when it's elevated for long periods of time, we get the message to STORE FAT. Additionally, lower levels of oestrogen change where our bodies deposit fat, shifting fat storage to our waists... and boom - a spare type appears, with many of us becoming increasingly apple-shaped. Great – just what you don't need in midlife as your confidence starts to wane!

It has been hypothesised that this is the cause of the middle-age spread; in all its wisdom, the female body wants to lay down some fat to produce some much-needed oestrogen (fat cells can make a type of oestrogen). The trouble is, none of us is that keen on weight gain as the solution for our depleted hormone levels! Interestingly, women with a body fat percentage of around 25% have fewer issues with osteoporosis, which is a consequence of low oestrogen. So, it's worth bearing in mind that a little extra padding does have its benefits. However, too much fat does the opposite!

> According to the American Journal of Clinical Nutrition women aged 40-59 should aim for a body fat percentage of 23-33% and women aged 60-79 slightly higher at 24-35%.

At this point, though, we shouldn't worry too much; just knowing about all this is empowering, because now we can adjust our way of eating, moving, and addressing our hormones to shift some weight – or prevent it going on in the first place. Just remember: it's never too late, no matter where you are on your journey. Knowledge is power!

Case study – Read Faye's Story

Meet Faye (Age 44)

Faye had had a total hysterectomy (uterus and ovaries

removed) in her 30s, and she came to me because, in her words, she had 'piled on the weight' even though she was exercising and following a strict diet (a mere 1000 calories a day!). She had lost her confidence and wasn't sure what to do next, as nothing seemed to shift the excess weight.

Faye was taking HRT to replace the hormones her body could no longer make, but – despite working out vigorously and eating very little to sustain herself – her diet wasn't working for her. She'd been advised to eat a low-calorie vegetarian diet and had ended up feeling utterly depleted. I suspected her cortisol levels were out of balance too. This pattern of living would have put a lot of strain on her body, and the strict dieting would have resulted in her losing muscle mass.

I started Faye on a healthy eating plan – which you'll learn about in this book – and, step by step, we changed her pattern of eating. This included having three meals a day (consisting of real foods, adequate amounts of protein, complex carbs, good fats, and greens – 'the feel-good four' food groups you're going to learn all about) and a 12-hour overnight fast. She placed less focus on cardio workouts and more on strength training, as well as giving herself more downtime for rest and relaxation.

Within three months, Faye was back down to her ideal weight – she was thrilled to have lost 10 kilos, and she also reported having more energy and enthusiasm for life!

The Transition

Everyone's transition is different. Perimenopause, for instance, is a bit like puberty, but in reverse. Remember when you were a stroppy teenager and your hormones were up and down like a yo-yo, but then you got a little older and things settled down? Of course, back then, the overall trend was that your hormones were on the way up.

For women like us, it's the same thing – with yo-yoing hormones – but the overall trend is that our hormones are ultimately on their way down.

It can be tempting at this point to reach for that extra glass of wine or to seek out comfort food in an attempt to make ourselves feel better, but sadly, these temporary fixes make us feel worse in the long run. However, if this is you, don't worry – you CAN break unhealthy habits, still have treats, and remain in control. This is what I'll help you with throughout this book: gaining motivation, instilling healthy habits, and taking things step by step.

Ring The Changes

Have a look at the symptoms body scan chart below and circle any symptoms that apply to you. It's surprising how many symptoms are actually related to perimenopause/menopause, plus, it's a useful exercise in terms of getting to know your body better and highlighting your symptoms.

Circle as appropriate

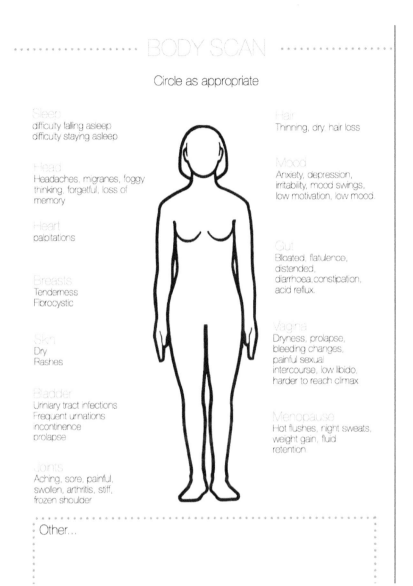

Sleep
difficulty falling asleep
difficulty staying asleep

Head
Headaches, migranes, foggy
thinking, forgetful, loss of
memory

Heart
palpitations

Breasts
Tenderness
Fibrocystic

Skin
Dry
Rashes

Bladder
Urinary tract infections
Frequent urinations
incontinence
prolapse

Joints
Aching, sore, painful,
swollen, arthritis, stiff,
frozen shoulder

Hair
Thinning, dry, hair loss

Mood
Anxiety, depression,
irritability, mood swings,
low motivation, low mood.

Gut
Bloated, flatulence,
distended,
diarrhoea, constipation,
acid reflux.

Vagina
Dryness, prolapse,
bleeding changes,
painful sexual
intercourse, low libido,
harder to reach climax

Menopause
Hot flushes, night sweats,
weight gain, fluid
retention

Other...

This hormone deficiency can really creep up on you, so let's explore the solutions and see what works for you.

CHAPTER 2 ~ FEEL GOOD ABOUT HORMONES

A Balanced Approach

Before we delve into diet and lifestyle, I think it would be remiss of me not to mention hormones. So, let's have a look at the pros and cons of taking hormone replacement therapy (HRT).

Why Would You Even Consider HRT?

A lot of women I talk to believe that HRT is taken purely to alleviate temporary symptoms like hot flushes and night sweats; what they don't realise is that it can protect you from debilitating diseases later in life, such as type 2 diabetes, osteoporosis, and heart disease. There is even some evidence that it can reduce your risk of dementia.

Nevertheless, as there's so much confusion and misinformation out there, I urge you to park your current beliefs – if you have any (I certainly did) – and read on.

I felt the need to address the subject in this book because, whilst diet and lifestyle are crucial and the bedrock of a healthy menopause, a hormone deficiency does have a significant impact on your body.

Therefore, whilst I'm not wishing to take the place of a medical expert in any way, what I am aiming to do is highlight the evidence both for and against HRT in order to give you a better understanding of this therapy.

HRT isn't for everyone, of course – it's such a personal choice – but please bear in mind that, for some women, the minor risks of taking it are outweighed by the many benefits.

I appreciate that some of you reading this may have other reasons why you can't take HRT, perhaps due to a family history of breast cancer, or because you've had breast or some other form of cancer. In this case, I urge you to look at the latest information available, see the resources section, and focus on the many areas of diet and lifestyle that can really make a difference to your body.

And do remember, there are post-menopause women who don't take HRT and who remain happy and healthy. Here, maybe we can learn from our Asian counterparts and focus on real foods that are rich in fibre, phytoestrogens, and quality proteins, as well as nourishing, supportive lifestyles. More on that later.

My Experience Of HRT

Up until a year ago, I was determined that I wouldn't be one of those women who relied on HRT to live my life – plus, surely, it was too big a risk for breast cancer. I was also of the opinion, like many women, that because I followed a healthy lifestyle, I probably wouldn't experience many symptoms and that I'd be able to tough it out – forever the optimist! I also regarded taking HRT as a sign of weakness; I preferred to be 'au naturel' and free from any medication.

My opinion and decision to avoid HRT at all costs, then – just like many others – had been shaped by the fear of getting breast cancer. Surely, menopause is just a natural process – we just need to get through it, and tough it out. Right?

What's Wrong With HRT?

Let's consider what drives the scary breast cancer headlines that stop many of us from even considering HRT in the first place.

The news that HRT increases your risk of breast cancer came from a study published in 2002, which alarmed women and doctors alike. It got us all thinking that HRT was to be avoided at all costs. It gave the impression that HRT and breast cancer were synonymous.

The study in question was conducted by the Women's Health Initiative (WHI). It was a large randomised controlled observational study (the most respected kind of scientific study) that followed 161,000 women, over seven to eight years, who were either taking HRT or a placebo.

The study concluded that HRT significantly increased a woman's risk of breast cancer and heart disease – which resulted in the study being stopped prematurely – and these findings, of course, made headline news. Many women were told to stop taking HRT, and women coming up to menopausal age were discouraged from starting it in the first place.

It is now widely understood, however, that this study's conclusions were both widely flawed and misreported.

A Brief Explanation – Why Was It Flawed?

First, let's consider the women participating in this study: they were mostly in their mid-60s, 50% were smokers or past smokers, 70% were overweight or obese, and a third had been treated for high blood pressure.

This is important, because smoking and being overweight are both much bigger stand-alone risk factors for breast cancer and cardiovascular disease than taking HRT (see info below)! Therefore, it wasn't at all representative of a typical healthy woman starting HRT, usually between the ages of 45 and 55.

However, this flawed reporting was BIG news and many women stopped taking their HRT overnight (and suffered the consequences). Understandably, after this study, doctors also became reluctant to prescribe it.

I recall one of the first ladies who found her way to my clinic many years ago, telling me how frustrated she was that her doctor wouldn't allow her to continue her HRT. She was in her mid-60s and had been taking it for over a decade. I was struck by just how upset she was; she told me that her mood was low, she had started suffering from aches and pains, she felt very tired in general, and she didn't enjoy her life anymore. How awful! At the time, I had no idea why this was. Now that I fully understand the role hormones play, I get why she felt so bereft at having her HRT withdrawn so suddenly.

This study has since been reanalysed, and it has been determined that the findings were not accurate; the risks of breast cancer and heart disease were not significantly increased by the women taking HRT in comparison to their lifestyle factors – such as alcohol intake, smoking, or being overweight. However, its legacy of misleading information lives on!

Professor Robert Langer, one of the original investigators of the Women's Health Initiative, has admitted that errors in this 2002 study led to a lot of unnecessary suffering for women who were encouraged to give up their HRT overnight.

Unfortunately, this U-turn didn't make the headlines and is not a well-known fact! What a shame for all women – especially as it's estimated that a third of women in the UK are either perimenopausal or menopausal. That's approximately 13 million of us.

Of course, what most of us are worried about is taking HRT and increasing our risk of breast cancer. So, let's get informed!

Both the NHS and NICE (the National Institute for Health and Care Excellence) state that the risks associated with HRT are small and are usually outweighed by the benefits.

According to NICE – the institute responsible for informing the NHS which drugs and treatments are safe and efficacious – the stats are as follows.

If you take 1000 healthy women between the ages of 50 and 59 and observe their health for five years, this is what you'll find. Bear with me; this is worth knowing!

- 23 of the 1000 women will get breast cancer – that's just the way it is. Sadly, our risk of breast cancer increases as we get older.
- An additional five women will get breast cancer if they drink two units of alcohol per night. That's one glass of wine, for example – not much, is it?
- Another 4-10 women will get breast cancer if they are overweight or obese.
- Another four women will get breast cancer if they take combined HRT (oestrogen and progesterone).

As you can see, drinking alcohol daily and being overweight are bigger risk factors for breast cancer than taking HRT.

Davina McCall demonstrated this well in the Channel 4 documentary, *Sex, Myths and*

the Menopause – in a ball pit of all places! If you haven't already seen it, it's worth catching up on.

NICE also states that any woman over the age of 45 who is suffering with menopausal symptoms is entitled to HRT.

I'm also including a chart here to reiterate this information:

Difference in breast cancer incidence per 1000 women aged 50-59

Approximate number of women developing breast cancer over the next five years

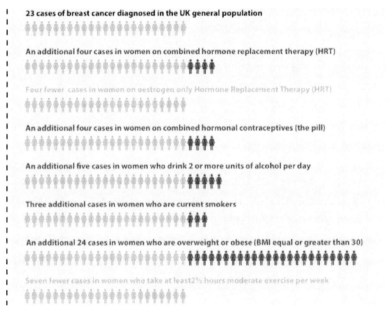

Women's Health Concern NICE Guideline, Menopause: Diagnosis and Management November 2015 (https://thebms.org.uk/wp-content/uploads/2016/04/WHC-UnderstandingRisksofBreastCancer-MARCH2017.pdf)

What Else May Have Made a Difference?

Additionally, the type of HRT used in the WHI study was different to the HRT that is typically prescribed today.

One such form of HRT used was Premarin, which is short for pregnant mares' urine (Pre mar in), and which is basically conjugated horse oestrogen! This was commonly prescribed at the time.

Some women in the study were taking this form of oestrogen, which has a different molecular structure to the oestrogen we naturally produce – which is known as bioidentical or body identical oestrogen.

What Are Bioidentical Hormones Aka Body Identical Hormones?

Basically, these are man-made hormones, created from yams and soy, which are formed of identical molecules to those we produce ourselves. Studies show that these preparations are safer for women than more traditional preparations, and they're also available on the NHS!

Therefore, as well as the cohort of women in the WHI study being atypical (that is, they were older than the average age of women typically starting HRT), they also had other independent risk factors for breast cancer and heart disease. On top of this, the type of HRT used wasn't as safe as the forms that are recommended by most doctors today.

Now let's look at oestrogen replacement. In the WHI study oestrogen was taken orally, but we now know there's a small risk of clotting when taken orally; the more modern forms of oestrogen, therefore, are prescribed as patches or gels to be applied directly to the skin. Taken in this form, there's no risk of clotting because when oestrogen is given topically via the skin, it doesn't pass through the liver, and the clotting risk is removed.

In some of those earlier studies, the replacement pro-gesterone was also in a synthetic form – again, a different molecular structure to what our bodies naturally make. It is now widely accepted that a safer option is micronised progesterone, which goes under the name of Utrogestan in the UK.

Therefore, whilst HRT does bring with it a small risk of breast cancer, by understanding this information and the context of the study, you can better put all the risks into perspective and make your own decision about taking HRT. Ask yourself – does the small risk outweigh the benefits for you as an individual?

For more information on what types of HRT are bioidentical, do look at: https://www.balance-menopause.com/menopause-library/hrt-the-different-ingredients-brands-and-strengths-available/

Alcohol in Menopause

A lot of women tell me they look forward to a drink during the perimenopause because it cheers them up and dampens their anxiety, yet they struggle with energy or motivation to exercise and are more likely to comfort eat.

Let's say you do take HRT and, consequently, you have more energy and are able to do more exercise, you lose some weight, have less cravings and become less dependent on alcohol – then it may be that you're lowering your risk of breast cancer and putting the odds in your favour!

Everything in life has a risk attached to it; understanding yours and deciding what's right for you is surely the best way to approach it.

Pros And Cons

So, what are the benefits of HRT? Why even take this small risk of breast cancer?

For one thing, HRT remains the most effective scientifically proven treatment for menopausal symptoms.

In short, not only can HRT get rid of the many symptoms associated with menopause – such as low mood, hot flushes, anxiety, brain fog, depression, vaginal issues, and insomnia – it can also protect your future health.

Protecting Your Future Health

Bones

Oestrogen is needed to help form new bone and this explains why women lose bone mass at menopause. Age UK estimates that one in two women after the age of 50 will break a bone at some point due to osteoporosis, (porous/fragile bones). Taking oestrogen during the menopause can help protect our bones and may prevent this from happening. See the chapter on bones for advice on how to take care of yours.

> My lovely grandmother had a hysterectomy in her mid-40s and suffered from crippling osteoporosis in her later years – if only I'd known then what I know now! With very little oestrogen in her body from her mid-40s onwards, there would have been little chance of her maintaining strong bones.

Heart health

Heart disease is one of the leading causes of death in women in the UK after menopause. The risk of heart and cardio-vascular disease increases at menopause and as our oestrogen drops off, at which point our risk catches up with that of men. HRT reduces our risk significantly if taken before the age of 60.

Diabetes

At menopause, our risk of type 2 diabetes increases. This is because the decline in oestrogen makes us less sensitive to insulin which has a detrimental effect on our blood sugar levels, hence we need to pay more attention to our diets.

Brain health

The brain is very sensitive to oestrogen, so when oestrogen declines, women's brains suffer; brain fog is a common complaint for women, and it doesn't stop there. Oestrogen is a neuro-protective hormone – it encourages new cell growth, it protects cells against damage, and it ensures that our neurons keep firing and that our brain cells continue to form new connections, thus keeping brain fog, brain damage, and memory loss at bay. Oestrogen can also affect our serotonin levels, which can impact how happy we feel. This explains why a lot of women feel less relaxed and confident during menopause.

This deficit in oestrogen may explain why dementia and Alzheimer's are the leading cause of death in the UK for women since 2011– who knew! The Alzheimer's Society states that twice as many women suffer from dementia as men.

Evidence shows that the earlier you start taking HRT, the more protection your brain will have; the advice is to take it within the first 10 years of menopause.

I'd urge you to read Lisa Mosconi's groundbreaking book, *The XX Brain*, which empowers women to prevent dementia.

Colon cancer

A lower risk of colon cancer is also associated with taking HRT.

In summary, more recent studies show that women who take HRT live longer and feel better, both physically and mentally. If you'd like to read more about why oestrogen is so important, check out *Oestrogen Matters* by oncologist Dr Avrum Bluming & Carol Tavris. This extensive, well-researched book looks at the evidence around the safety of oestrogen and concludes that: "Women's lives can be improved without increasing their risk of breast cancer."

There are also some great podcasts on the subject that are much lighter than the book, and a good starting point for anyone wanting to find out more. Liz Earle discusses this topic extensively in her podcast, *The Liz Earle Wellbeing Show* – a good episode to check out is her conversation with Professor Michael Baum.

Another fantastic resource is the website Balance Menopause, which is a comprehensive, evidence-based resource for understanding HRT and menopause. The founder, Louise Newson, is a medical doctor and menopause specialist, and is such a champion for women and their right to access replacement hormones. She's been brave enough to challenge the authoritative voices that have argued against her, and she's still going strong, getting her message and scientifically proven information out there while helping women the length and breadth of the country! You can find out more at the following links:

https://www.balance-menopause.com

https://www.themenopausecharity.org

These sites will give you a well-referenced and up-to-date source of studies supporting the use of oestrogen and HRT in general, should you wish to find out more.

The NHS and NICE (National Institute for Health and Care

Excellence) state that the risks associated with HRT are small and are usually outweighed by its benefits.

In general, HRT can help with the following symptoms:

Hot flushes, night sweats, irregular periods, mood swings, vaginal dryness, low libido, headaches, breast soreness, burning mouth, joint pains, digestive issues, bloating, electric shock sensations, sore muscles, gum issues, tingling in extremities, fatigue, itchy skin, anxiety, disrupted sleep, hair loss, brain fog, difficulty concentrating, weight gain, dizzy spells, stress incontinence, brittle nails, allergies, palpitations, irritability, body odour, depression and low mood, and osteoporosis.

If you wish to explore HRT, you absolutely should; there really is no need to feel embarrassed or timid. You have the right to get the help you need. Remember, in the UK, menopause is happening right now to 13 million of us – so you're in good company!

The Cons

Yes, there is a slight increase in the risk of breast cancer. NICE states that there is no increase if taking oestrogen only – however, you'd only do this if you've had your uterus removed. For women with a uterus, progesterone is needed to prevent endometrial hyperplasia, that is, a build-up of the lining of the womb that can lead to womb cancer. Hence, for most of us, it's necessary to take oestrogen and progesterone together.

And, remember, if you take HRT and continue to drink every night, remain inactive, and stay overweight, then you're increasing your risk of breast cancer significantly. Therefore, you really want to manage the odds and put them in your favour.

Some women feel that HRT isn't working for them when they first start taking it, but do bear in mind that with this – as with many treatments – a personalised approach is often required. For instance, if your dose is wrong or if the type of HRT doesn't suit you, don't be afraid to speak up; your health and wellbeing are definitely worth the time and effort to get it right.

Some doctors are still reluctant to prescribe HRT, although most are becoming better informed as menopause is being taken more seriously. However, it's always worth being informed and empowered to make your own case. When seeing your GP, make a list of your symptoms and explain why you think HRT might help. Be persistent, and continue with your queries until you find a doctor that can help.

Taking HRT

Of course, some women don't want to take any medication at all, preferring instead the more natural alternatives, but do bear in mind that whilst herbs such as black cohosh and sage may help reduce your symptoms of hot flushes, they won't protect your bones or your heart health. In this case, you'll have to focus on your diet and exercise to give yourself the very best chance of avoiding issues later in life.

A Personalised Approach

Whilst we've all heard stories of GPs refusing to give women HRT, or offering up antidepressants instead, there seems to be a sea change; many doctors are working very hard to change all this, by educating healthcare providers on the effects of menopause.

Unfortunately, menopausal issues are still woefully neglected within the NHS, but this too is changing.

Remember: the NICE guidelines clearly state that any woman over the age of 45 who is suffering from menopausal symptoms is entitled to HRT on the NHS. So don't be afraid to ask.

Taking HRT is a personal choice, but no matter your reasons, it's sensible to consider your options and weigh up your personal pros and cons so that you can make a well-informed decision with your healthcare professional – a decision that suits you, and only you.

How to approach a visit to the GP to discuss HRT:

1. When making an appointment at your GP surgery, ask if there's a GP who has an interest in women's health or menopause.

2. Make a list of your symptoms to take with you (see body scan) or anything you think may be related.

3. Give a description of what your last year's periods have entailed – heavy, light, short or long cycles, spotting, painful?

4. If you're told you're too young, too old, or simply not suitable for HRT, ask to be referred to an NHS menopause clinic.

Think Of It Like This

Some doctors think of menopause as a hormone deficiency.

If you have diabetes, then your doctor is going to prescribe insulin. If you have an underactive thyroid, you're going to take thyroxine to replace this missing hormone. You may say to yourself: is it natural to take hormones? Is it what nature intended? No, but then neither is taking thyroxine or insulin. Despite this, we use modern science to our advantage on a daily basis – so that we can live our best, healthiest lives. We're not much use to ourselves – or others – if we're going about our days as angry, tired, anxious, unhappy insomniacs.

It's also useful to reflect on the fact that we live a lot longer these days. In Victorian times, the average life span of a woman was somewhere between 57 to 59 years of age. In modern times, most of us can expect to live for another three decades after menopause.

> Queen Victoria was the exception; she lived to the grand old age of 81 and was reported to have a waist measuring 50 inches – there's always an outlier! She did look a bit miserable though :(

If you're interested, here's a bit more background information on hormones – if you're not, you can just move on to the next chapter.

Whistle-stop Tour – Get To Know Your Hormones Better

Oestrogen

We think of oestrogen as being one single hormone but, in fact, we produce three different types:

Oestrone (E1)

Made mainly in fat tissue, we tend to make more of this type as we get older. Larger amounts of this one are associated with inflammation and an increased risk of breast cancer.

Oestradiol (E2) – The Diva Hormone

This hormone gives us our feminine curves (think of it as the Diva Hormone). It plays a role in building bones, contributes to our brain health, reduces our LDL cholesterol (the less desirable type) and increases our HDL (the good type), helps our skin to make and retain collagen, and makes us less insulin resistant and less likely to gain weight. Most HRT preparations use this type of oestrogen.

Oestriol (E3)

This is the weakest form of oestrogen. We tend to produce high levels of this during pregnancy.

Symptoms of low oestrogen include: anxiety, bone loss, brain fog, dry skin, dry eyes, depression, headaches, hot flushes, insomnia, low libido, palpitations, thinning hair, vaginal dryness, and memory loss.

Also, recent research has shown that postmenopausal women are more likely to suffer more severely from Covid-19, so optimal levels of oestrogen may help here too.

Progesterone

The Latin origin of this name is 'pro-gestation', meaning it grows the lining of the womb to support a pregnancy. It usually drops off first due to a lack of viable eggs (progesterone is made from the corpus luteum, so remember, no ovulation = no/low progesterone). Basically, it calms everything down – think of it as oestrogen's calming best friend!

Low levels of progesterone – what most of us experience initially with perimenopause – are often felt in our 40s.

Symptoms of low progesterone include: anxiety, abdominal pain, fatigue, irritability, insomnia, low libido, breast tenderness, spotting between periods, irregular periods, shorter cycles, low libido, headaches, and migraines.

Testosterone

This can make us feel 'sexy and confident', though I heard one doctor say that too much can make us 'sweaty and sleazy'! It's all about balance.

Half of our testosterone is made in our ovaries and our adrenal glands. We produce four times as much testosterone as we do oestrogen, though we tend to think of it as a male hormone only. Men, however, don't have a monopoly on it – it's just that we make it in much smaller amounts than they do. It's important for our libido and our ability to orgasm, it helps maintain our muscle strength, it affects our cognitive function, and it helps with motivation and mood.

Symptoms of low testosterone include: anxiety, hot flushes, low libido, weight gain, poor memory, reduced stamina, poor concentration, low energy, and depression.

There is, of course, a lot of overlap when it comes to hormone deficiencies. This list is certainly not extensive, and there may be other reasons why you're experiencing these symptoms.

You're The Custodian Of Your Own Health

I always point out to my clients that **no one is as invested in your health as you are**. Not your doctor, not your husband, not your nutritional therapist – just YOU. So, make sure you don't take this responsibility lightly. Be the custodian of your own health; no one else is going to do it for you.

Need To Know

Most of us experience many symptoms as our sex hormones drop off. If you're considering taking hormones, ensure you take body identical ones – also known as bioidentical – as these are available on the NHS.

Your medical expert can guide you with all of this, of course, but doing some homework before going to see them can really help. Here are some useful websites:

Balance Menopause – https://www.balance-menopause.com/

The British Menopause Society – https://thebms.org.uk/

The Menopause Charity – https://www.themenopausecharity.org/

When it comes to oestrogen, it is safest when taken topically – that is, via the skin in the form of a patch or a gel.

Progesterone can be taken orally as micronised progesterone (product name Utrogestan), as it has the same hormonal structure that we produce naturally. It's made from soy and yams but is highly regulated in the UK. In terms of developing breast cancer, it has a lower risk associated with it compared to its synthetic cousins. Some doctors prescribe the Mirena coil, which is a synthetic form of progesterone; it provides a very small, localised dose, and some women do better with this.

You should also be aware that progesterone is sold online as a cream, and you can easily find it on the internet. Please note that these products are not regulated by the Medicine and Healthcare Products Regulatory Agency (MHRA), so you have no assurance in terms of dose or quality. These, therefore, should be avoided.

Testosterone is more difficult to get prescribed on the NHS as, typically, the only testosterone product licensed in the UK is for use by men and delivers a much larger dose than is needed for women. There's an Australian brand called AndroFeme, though it's unlicensed in the UK so you'll have to try to persuade your doctor to prescribe it.

Testosterone can improve energy, libido, motivation, mood, and vaginal issues. I've observed doctors prescribing oestrogen and progesterone for the first three to six months and then, if a woman is still experiencing low libido or any of the above, they may well consider testosterone.

Final Thoughts

It's not my aim to persuade you to take hormones; rather, it's my goal to inform you of the choices that are available to YOU – plus, I wanted to dispel the belief that oestrogen is all bad and causes breast cancer. Of course, you may read this and be confident in your decision to remain HRT-free and look for other ways to support your menopause, and that might well be the right decision for you. The information here is purely to give you a brief understanding of HRT and is not intended to be a substitute for medical advice.

The rest of this book will focus on the countless other advantages you can give yourself to live a long and happy life beyond your 40s.

CHAPTER 3 ~ FEEL GOOD ABOUT EATING

Midlife is a time to nourish ourselves. Our bodies are dealing with a lot of change and will adjust to new normal, therefore it's essential that we focus on foods that sustain us and that we eat in a way that supports stable blood sugar levels.

> The word 'diet' stems from the Greek word DIAITA, meaning a way of life that supports health!

Let's Keep It Simple

Firstly, I'm going to familiarise you with **the feel-good four method.**

This method is simply a guide to help you find the best sources of protein, fats, carbohydrates, and greens. It also ensures your plate has all the food types your body requires without you having to weigh everything or worry about calories. It will help you feel energised and satiated, and it will reduce cravings for sugary foods – which is vital if you want to stay well! It will also provide you with the nutrients you'll need as you transition through menopause.

So, when it comes to food, we need to look at **quality over quantity** every time – this will really help regulate your appetite and your health. Therefore, I encourage you to ditch processed foods and reach for healthier, unadulterated foods. Soon, you'll be reaping the benefits.

The Feel-Good Four Equals the Feel-Good You

This is such a great concept, especially as it's so simple to use when putting a meal together. You just need to ensure that your plate has the feel-good four on it – that is:

PROTEIN, GOOD CARBS, FATS, AND SOME GREENS.

At this stage of our lives, it's important that we pay more attention to what we eat, so we can give our body the nourishment it needs to flourish and age in a healthful way. Eating the feel-good four will ensure we do just that – without overcomplicating things.

We'll look at the importance of all these food groups in more detail shortly, but just to say that this way of eating really suits midlife women; it ensures we're covering all the bases from a nutritional standpoint. Cleansing, detoxing, and deprivation is not where it's at!

So, let's look at each component of the feel-good four in more depth:

Protein – this helps us with blood sugar control, which in turn helps us maintain a healthy weight. It helps contribute to our muscles and bones, allowing us to stay strong. Protein also decreases our hunger hormones so we're more likely to feel full. Research indicates that by eating approximately 20-30g of protein in the morning, you will be supporting your blood sugar balance and will be less likely to overeat later in the day. Additionally, as we get older it's harder for the body to absorb protein, therefore it's more important than ever that we have adequate amounts.

Good carbs (meaning unadulterated/fibre-rich carbohydrates) – these keep us fuller for longer, help balance our blood sugar, contribute to a healthy gut, prevent constipation, and lower our risk of disease. We really want to upgrade our carbs, rather than avoid them altogether.

Fats – these turn off hunger hormones, fill us up, and help us absorb critical vitamins like A, D, E, and K. Plus, fat is a good source of essential fatty acids. Fat also provides us with the raw materials we need to make hormones, and it's a great carrier of flavour too.

Greens – these provide us with a rich array of vitamins, minerals, and plant compounds that have major benefits to the body in terms of reducing the risk of disease, plus they contribute to bone and heart health. They're also some of the most nutrient-dense foods we can put into our bodies.

So, all you need to do is focus on the feel-good four when putting a meal together. Simply ask yourself: Does this meal contain the feel-good four? Just check off each food group as you put them on your plate. Let's look at each one in more detail:

PROTEIN

You're aiming for 20-30g of protein per meal – see the chapter on protein for advice on quantities by food type.

Good sources of protein include:

Fish – salmon, sardines, smoked salmon, mackerel, haddock, hake, cod

Seafood – crab, mussels, prawns, scallops

Meats – venison, beef, lamb, pork (no more than once/twice a week)

Poultry – chicken, turkey

Vegetarian sources:

Legumes – beans, chickpeas, lentils

Soya – tofu, tempeh

Nuts and seeds – almonds, cashews, pecans, walnuts, pumpkin seeds, sunflower seeds, hemp seeds

Quinoa

Eggs

(Legumes are healthy sources of both protein and good carbs – see the protein chapter for more guidance on quantities.)

And, if you eat meat and fish, I'd recommend aiming for at least a minimum of a couple of plant-based days a week; there is mounting evidence that a highly plant-based diet is associated with longevity and lesser risks of all the major diseases. There is also some evidence to suggest that a more plant-based diet dampens the symptoms of menopause – and, of course, it's better for animals and our oceans!

"Even when we can't do everything, we can do something" – Simon Reeve.

GOOD COMPLEX CARBS

What we're looking for here is good unadulterated carbohydrates, leaving the stripped grains like flour and processed beige foods behind; for most of us, this will result in a spike in our blood sugar, and after the high always comes the low – which results in cravings. Exactly what we don't want!

In terms of quantities, think approximately a quarter to a half of your plate – or more like half if your complex carbs are coming from just vegetables.

Some women at this stage avoid carbohydrates altogether, but I don't believe this is necessary. Upgrading your carbohydrates and getting the quantities in check is a far better approach.

Familiarise yourself with the carbohydrate pyramid below so you can make the best choices.

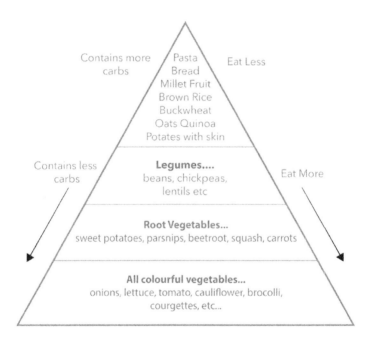

Amanda Ryder

You can base your carbohydrate choices around these:

Vegetables – opt for lots of colour. I include them here, although some – like peppers, for example – will contain a lot less carbs

Legumes – remember, these contain protein and carbs

Lentils

Beans – all types

Chickpeas

Root vegetables – sweet potatoes, carrots with skin, white potatoes with skin or cold potatoes, squash, beetroot, celeriac, parsnips

Brown rice, basmati, black rice

Quinoa

Buckwheat

Oats

Chia seeds – these are a good choice as almost half their weight is fibre

Flaxseed

Whole spelt, whole wheat, spelt, barley

> Vegetables that are grown below ground, such as root veg, tend to have more carbohydrates than vegetables grown above ground, like broccoli, cauliflower, peppers etc. However, legumes have more carbohydrates than all vegetables but usually less than grains.

Why?

When I say 'good complex carbohydrates', I just mean carbohydrates that have a complex structure and contain more fibre. These types of carbohydrates take longer to hit the bloodstream in the form of blood glucose and help us avoid a blood sugar spike. We'll look at why they're better for us in the next chapter.

If you don't eat any carbohydrates at all and tend to base your diet around proteins, with just vegetables or salads on the side, you may find that you're often irritable and don't sleep as well. Carbohydrates are often demonised and blamed for weight gain, but often, it's simply because people are eating too many processed carbohydrates. However, if you can focus on the good complex kind, then a couple of portions daily can be very beneficial to your health.

Good carbs – eaten along with protein and fat – can help stabilise blood sugar and energy levels, feed your gut bugs, and improve your mood. The trick is not to eat them on their own.

Note: Remember that sweet potatoes, carrots, beetroot, and all veg that grow under the ground contain carbs but a lot less than grains, making them an excellent choice for a midlife woman.

> Potatoes get a bad rap, but cold potatoes are an excellent source of good complex carbs. This is because – once they've been cooked and cooled – they make a fibre called resistant starch. Why not keep some cooked potatoes in the fridge and then sauté them in olive oil? (Fortunately, reheating them doesn't remove this fibre.) Then you'll have your good carbs.

So, your choices of good carbs for the day might look like:

- Some oats and flaxseed for breakfast with a piece of fruit
- Lentil or chickpea salad for lunch with a piece of fruit
- Sweet potato wedges in the evening, or
- Brown rice and steamed vegetables, or
- Potato wedges and roasted vegetables.

FAT

Your fats can include:

Olive oil
Avocados
Coconut oil
Butter
Tahini
Nuts
Seeds
Nut butter – almond, peanut etc.
Oily fish*
* An average size fillet of wild Alaskan salmon contains 6 grams of essential healthy fats.

Why Do We Need Fats?

Not only do fats help our bodies function better, but they are also a great carrier of flavour.

Fats provide us with the raw ingredients to make hormones, absorb our fat-soluble vitamins, support our brain, and keep our skin hydrated and radiant.

I'm not against all saturated fats – such as butter, red meat, and cheese – however, I'd recommend that you only enjoy them from time to time and, instead, prioritise unsaturated fats like olive oil and fats found in nuts, seeds, avocados, and oily fish. The evidence is clear – these types of fat are much better for our health.

GREENS

These can include:

Broccoli
Rocket
Cabbage
Watercress
Kale
Spinach
Chard
Fresh herbs
Lettuce
Lamb's lettuce
Romaine lettuce
Pak choi
Green peas

Why?

There are many, many benefits to eating greens. They contain powerful chemicals that protect our bodies against disease, they supply us with myriad vitamins, minerals, and fibre, they help support the body's detoxification process to help rid ourselves of unwanted toxins, and they support our bone health. They also contain plenty of the (mighty!) magnesium that's needed for energy, bone health, blood sugar control, blood pressure control, and many other vital functions throughout the body.

Putting All This Into Practise

So, now you know all this, you need to get into the habit of asking yourself: Is this meal going to give me **the feel-good four?**

It may seem like a lot of changes – or not, depending on where you are with your diet. In the next few sections, I'm going to give you some background info. and inspiration on why this concept really works, but for now, all YOU need to do is focus on getting those feel-good four onto your plate for most of your meals.

Did you know that when approaching your meal, it's a good idea to eat your vegetables first and then your protein, followed by your fats and carbohydrates. This results in less of a blood sugar spike, which has a huge impact on your health going forward. More on this later.

I'm keen to get you started so that you can feel the benefits straight away. So, have a look at the table below and mimic their ratios when it comes to your own foods. And don't worry – it doesn't have to be an exact science, just an overarching structure to your meals.

The Feel-Good Four Meal Examples

Most days, aim to include the feel-good four in two to three meals.

I've included vegetables under the good carbs banner to keep it simple, but things like peppers and tomatoes (technically a fruit) can also be included here. Do aim for as much variety as you can.

Here are some pointers:

- For one portion of protein, use the size of your palm as an approximate measure.
- Make sure that a quarter to a half of your plate is filled with good carbs – colourful vegetables, legumes, sweet potatoes – and if having grains, like rice, oats, pasta, then make it more like a 1/4 of your plate.

- For one portion of greens, use either a good handful, a cup, or a quarter of your plate as a guideline.
- For fats, use 1-2 tbsp (some fats will be found in protein, like oily fish/eggs).
- Include a piece of fruit either after or with your meal.

Start by trying out the recipes in this book and, gradually, you'll get the hang of it. There is, of course, lots of overlap – for instance, a lot of foods such as legumes contain carbohydrates and protein, whereas fish, eggs, and meat contain protein and fats – but as you read through, you'll become better at identifying these. And, of course, you can just follow the recipes and mimic the ratios in your own creations. This is just a rough guide and doesn't need to be exact.

| Most of the recipes in this book include the feel-good four |

What you are aiming for with your meals is something like this – it doesn't have to be a recipe.

Feel-Good Four Meal Examples

Protein	Complex carbs	Greens	Fats
2/3 eggs cooked to your liking	1 piece of sourdough or rye bread with mushrooms and tomatoes	sautéed spinach	½ an avocado
tofu stir-fry	brown rice veg such as peppers and spring onions	broccoli	olive oil

sautéed salmon	sweet potato wedges	steamed broccoli	tahini dressing
fillet of chicken or thigh	colourful tray of roasted veg	kale, or put something green in with roasted veg like broccoli	olive oil
smoked mackerel	a lentil salad with ½ an avocado, cucumber, and cherry tomatoes	rocket	tahini dressing
2 eggs	baked beans or 1 slice of sourdough or rye	½ an avocado or sautéed spinach	olive oil
full fat yoghurt	grated apple / a handful of berries	skip for this one	flax or chia seeds and nuts
chickpeas	chickpeas	rocket, avocado, lettuce, red onion & cherry tomato salad	olive oil, feta cheese
green smoothie, silken tofu, or protein powder	flaxseed	greens such as celery, spinach, or lettuce	tahini

There may be times when you don't have the greens, or the protein might be on the light side, but the reality of eating well is just getting it right most of the time. It's the 80:20 rule; because it's what we do regularly that makes the biggest difference.

What About Fruit?

Eat fruit like the Mediterranean's do – that is, as part of a meal – and aim for no more than three pieces of fruit daily. Get into the habit of enjoying a piece of fruit at the end of a meal; treat it like a dessert. If you're trying to lose weight, you may want to skip the fruit with your evening meal.

> Always eat your fruit – avoid drinking it in the form of juice! Once the fibre has been removed, juice just becomes a very concentrated form of sugar. If you want to enjoy juice now and again, dilute it with water – 50:50 – or sip it slowly with a meal to avoid the blood sugar spike. Slices of melon, a fruit salad, apples and blueberries, or a bowl of assorted berries served with some fresh mint and lime juice make a nice dessert.

What About Water?

Aim to drink 1-1.5 litres of water daily, in between meals; too much water with your meal may interfere with digestion. However, a glass of water before a meal can be helpful for weight regulation. I encourage my clients to drink a glass of water before breakfast, lunch, and dinner because it suppresses a hormone called vasopressin.

> When our bodies detect that we're dehydrated, we produce more vasopressin, and high levels of vasopressin are found in overweight individuals. This is because this hormone conserves water in the body – which can ultimately lead to weight gain, as the body is encouraged to store fat as part of this process. Staying hydrated, therefore, can be helpful for all of us and will contribute to better weight regulation.

A good habit to get into is to fill a jug of water first thing in the morning and have it somewhere you can see it – this way, you'll be reminded to drink it! Add mint and cucumber or lemons and limes to make it more enticing. Mild dehydration can often be mistaken for hunger, which is why it's a good idea to drink a glass of water before heading to the fridge.

Eating like this is hugely beneficial. We make bad decisions when we're very hungry, and this way of eating does away with cravings. However, as you transition to this new way of eating – that is, with the structure of two / three meals a day and less snacking – you may feel hungry initially. In most cases, just four or five days of eating like this are all it takes to get you and your blood sugar on an even keel and working in your favour.

Organise Your Fridge

If you can make your environment healthier, then it's much easier to make good choices. I find a well-organised fridge is one way of doing this. For example, make sure you have things such as olives, pre-cooked greens like broccoli, sauerkraut and condiments, dips like hummus, crudités like chopped carrot batons, berries, mackerel pate (see recipe), and grapes all on the top shelf. Then, have another shelf dedicated to protein-rich foods such as tofu, fish, eggs, kefir, and coconut/dairy yoghurts. Finally, you can have another area filled with colourful vegetables, and a drawer or box full of greens such as rocket, spinach, and watercress – just make sure they're all in full sight!

So, you've got your fridge sorted, but what if you constantly find you're still hungry after a meal?

The Rule Of 20

Always give it at least 20 minutes after finishing a meal, and then decide if you really want or need more food. Why 20 minutes? Because that's the time it takes for our brains to get the message we're full. I'm sure we can all hold out for 20 minutes, but changing habits always requires some effort. Distract yourself, phone a friend, go for a walk, and just get out of the kitchen! It gets easier with time. Remember: prioritising later (your health further down the line if you don't overeat) over now (eating what you fancy all the time) always pays off!

And lastly, if you fancy something sweet, it's much better to have it at the end of your meal. Your diet is all about balance and making the right choices that suit you as an individual.

> Dark chocolate is an excellent choice. Not only does it taste good but it's rich in magnesium, iron, and antioxidants, and contributes to a healthy heart and blood pressure... which are all important at midlife. Don't overdo it, though; 2-4 small squares are enough.

You may have noticed that once we start to transition through menopause, our hormone levels fluctuate, which can have a massive impact on our appetite. That's why, one day, you feel like you're in total control, and the next you just want to snaffle up everything in sight.

Follow the advice here and – with time – you'll gain much more control over your appetite and, therefore, won't need to rely on your discipline and willpower alone to resist cravings. Your blood sugar control will become more stable so that when you do have a bad day, you'll just put it behind you and get back on track the next – after all, you're only human and none of us are able to completely resist forbidden treats!

Treats have their place, but they should be enjoyed now and again rather than every day.

Remember. ... **if you're not feeding the body with good quality, nourishing food, then make sure you're feeding the soul** – e.g. with something you really desire, like a delicious cake or whatever your favourite indulgence is. If you're not feeding either, then it's better to just give it a miss and move on!

My experience has taught me that when individuals completely restrict their favourite foods, they often crave and think about that food more than they ever did. Whereas, if they allow themselves to enjoy that treat now and again, their intense cravings disappear. Simply put, a little of what you fancy is OK; saying to yourself 'I'm never going to eat another chip or sugary treat ever again' is unrealistic.

So, now that you have an outline and structure for the way you eat, let's consider how to feel good about your weight.

CHAPTER 4 ~ FEEL GOOD ABOUT YOUR WEIGHT (AND GET GOOD AT CARBS)

Before we consider the benefits of the feel-good four food groups in more detail, let's drill down on what we can do to avoid weight gain and keep ourselves healthy. I'll also show you the problem with yo-yo dieting and how to avoid common mistakes when it comes to staying on top of your weight. Of course, you are more than your weight, but it's a common problem in midlife, and understanding why women can struggle with maintaining their weight is useful going forward.

There are two main hormones that we can – and will – influence with diet and lifestyle: **insulin** and **cortisol**. First, let's look at what we can do to keep insulin in check, as well as consider other factors that contribute to weight gain and what we can do about them.

Why Am I Gaining Weight?

One of the main reasons a lot of us start to gain weight at midlife is because we have lower levels of oestrogen, which is compounded by the fact that a lot of us will have lower muscle mass compared to when we were younger. At this stage, for a lot of us, our once steady body composition starts to shift.

As our oestrogen declines, we don't handle carbohydrates as well as we did before – our cells are less sensitive to insulin, hence we don't get away with treats as easily as we once did. As a result, we tend to put on weight around our middle –

frustrating! On top of this, our metabolism also slows down; it's estimated that we burn 200 fewer calories per day at this stage of our lives.

Pre-menopausal levels of oestrogen ensured that our bodies were sensitive to insulin (the hormone that helps regulate blood sugar), so at that point, our blood sugar levels were easier to maintain. However, when there's less oestrogen around, it becomes much harder to maintain what feels like a stable weight.

Therefore, to avoid this scenario, we really do have to pay attention to our carbohydrates, upgrading from the white, processed, mainly beige variety, to the health-giving, good, complex, colourful kind.

If you follow the advice here, you can still eat great-tasting food, assert control over what you put in your mouth, and avoid what might seem like the inevitable weight gain... yes, it can be done!

An underactive thyroid can exacerbate menopausal symptoms, and thyroid issues are more prevalent in midlife, which can lead to weight gain and other issues. Our thyroid gland is responsible for our metabolism, you can think of it as our thermostat – if it's on low, you won't be burning as much energy or functioning as well. The thyroid makes two hormones that all cells in our body require to function. So, if you're struggling with fatigue, constipation, hair loss, or unexplained weight gain, it may be worth getting your thyroid tested. Your doctor can test your TSH (thyroid-stimulating hormone) and T4 (thyroxine).

What's Muscle Got To Do With Weight?

Let's consider the loss of muscle mass. Muscle is a very metabolically active tissue, which just means it uses up a lot of calories, even at rest – so a good muscle mass equates to a faster metabolism. Think of it as your engine.

As we get into our 40s, we naturally tend to lose some of our muscle mass – this is known as sarcopenia. It's also been observed that a lot of midlife women are less active than their younger selves, and may be restricting calories because they're watching their weight. Unfortunately, all these things chip away at overall muscle mass.

Weight loss, unfortunately, often results in muscle loss too!

Less muscle = easier weight gain.

Therefore, it's so important that we do all we can to maintain our muscle mass by eating adequate amounts of protein (more on that later) and by finding a weight-bearing exercise we enjoy and that we can do on a regular basis – around 2/3 times a week.

Muscle Mass Is Critical Beyond Our 40s

Think of it like this: the more muscle you have, the bigger engine you have, and the more fuel/calories you'll burn, meaning...

Women with higher muscle mass have bigger engines, can eat more, and won't gain weight as easily.

Who doesn't want that?

Be a Ferrari, not a Fiat 500 ;)

If you drive to the corner shop in a Ferrari, you'll use a lot more fuel that you would in a Fiat 500, even though the distance driven is the same!

Recent research clearly demonstrates that good levels of muscle mass correlate with a healthier, longer life, and this is a much better predictor of reaching old age in good health than the previously used metric of overall body mass known as BMI (body mass index). So, it's not all about weight loss. If you consider our older folk who struggle to get up and out of a chair, it's usually due to a lack of muscle mass and overall strength. It's a case of 'use it or lose it'.

Why Yo-yo Dieting Never Works

Below is a very simple explanation of what may happen during weight loss – and this is often the outcome of yo-yo dieting.

Please bear in mind that we're not equal amounts of fat and muscle. However, what I wanted to demonstrate here – in this very simple table – is how we lose muscle mass when dieting, and why we regain weight more easily (as fat) when we stop.

Helen's weight before the 'diet'	Helen loses 2 stone on a crash diet	Helen stops 'diet' & regains weight
She weighs:	She now weighs:	And now she weighs:
10 stone	8 stone	10 stone
5 stone of muscle	4 stone of muscle	4 stone of muscle
5 stone of fat	4 stone of fat	**6 stone of fat**

As you can see, initially, Helen lost equal amounts of muscle and fat. However, when she stopped following the diet and regained the weight, she ended up with a much smaller muscle mass – aka 'engine' – plus, the weight she regained went on as fat. So, you can see why yo-yo diets are a disaster for most of us.

This example is an exaggeration, but it often happens to some degree to women who follow calorie restrictive diets. That is, they lose muscle mass and fat during the diet and, once they return to their normal eating patterns, they often regain the weight as fat. This then slows their metabolism, hence they struggle to burn calories as efficiently as they did before the diet.

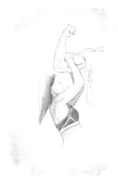

Therefore, you want to hang on to your muscle with all your might – because you don't want to slow down your metabolism, or compromise your strength or vitality, as you get older.

Additionally, good levels of muscle mass result in higher levels of testosterone.

During our 40s and 50s, we make a lot less testosterone – actually, it's estimated to be a mere half of what we had at our disposal in our 20s. Low levels of testosterone can also contribute to weight gain.

This is why incorporating some weight-bearing exercise into your life is a must (see chapter 14, where I discuss this in more detail).

> Weight-bearing exercises can help us make and maintain muscle, which is essential for bone health. Squats, lunges, lifting weights, walking up hills, walking with a weighted vest or rucksack, dancing, running, jumping, barre classes, yoga, pilates and gym classes like body pump are all strength-training exercises that can really help.

For now, let's focus on what we can do from a dietary perspective, including how to get our insulin in check. Remember: insulin regulates our blood sugar levels, and it's also involved in how our bodies store fat.

Why Are We Suddenly Focused on Insulin?

Our cells don't respond as well to insulin at midlife, hence we need to focus some attention here.

Think of it like this:

- Insulin is the key.
- Cell receptors are the locks to the doors.

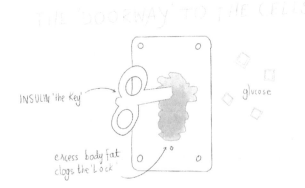

Insulin is the key that opens the lock for the glucose/blood sugar to move out of the bloodstream and into your cells.

When you have too much glucose in your bloodstream – say, after you've eaten a meal high in beige, processed carbohydrates, or sweet foods, or if you've been snacking all day long – it can result in high levels of blood sugar and, consequently, insulin.

This is something we really want to avoid, because insulin is a fat-storage hormone, and when it's elevated, it's telling your body to...

Store fat, store fat, store fat!

And remember where it's usually stored? That's right – around the middle!

Plus, fat around the middle can make us more prone to insulin resistance.

Chronically elevated insulin is a precursor to diabetes – which is the worst-case scenario, and something we want to avoid!

> Insulin is a hormone produced by the pancreas
>
> It's needed to take glucose from your blood and place it into your cells

So, let's consider what we can do to prevent this from happening.

Let's start with how to be competent at CARBS because most of us are on a blood sugar rollercoaster with dramatic highs and lows!

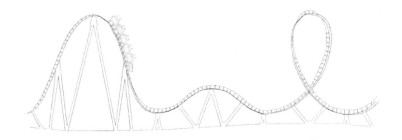

Let me explain the bedrock of all dietary principles – that is, the importance of balancing blood sugar. This just means how our bodies use and process glucose, which is present in all carbohydrates. Our blood sugar regulation has such a profound effect on how we feel, both physically and mentally, that it's of paramount importance when it comes to maintaining a good healthy weight and body. It's where I start with all my clients, so you'll really benefit from understanding this fully.

I've gone into detail here in my explanation of how we process carbohydrates because the women who are most successful in reaching their health goals are those who have a good grasp of how carbohydrates affect them. They understand that when blood sugar goes up quickly, insulin follows!

I find that many women in perimenopause and menopause have been advised to avoid carbohydrates altogether. However, this isn't necessary for most of us – or helpful when putting together a long-term healthy eating plan. For most of us, a life without any carbohydrates at all isn't easy or enjoyable. Plus, there are many benefits to including them in our diet. Therefore, it's far more important to focus on upgrading your carbohydrates and eating them as part of the feel-good four – and especially alongside protein.

So, how do we do this?

Firstly, it's important to understand that not all carbohydrates are created equal. However, they are all broken down in the body into a sugar known as blood glucose.

> Glucose is the body's preferred source of fuel, it comes from the food we eat and from our own body's stored glucose.

The time it takes your body to break down carbohydrates into glucose/blood sugar (the same thing) depends on which type of carbohydrate it is. It also depends on how much fibre it contains, or whether it's eaten alone or combined with other food groups such as protein, fibre and fats.

What we're aiming for is a slow release of glucose to avoid those blood sugar and insulin spikes that are so detrimental to our health and that can make menopause symptoms a lot worse!

The Best Order In Which To Eat Your Meal

Did you know that the order in which you eat your food can make all the difference to your blood sugar? Aim to eat your meal in this order to avoid blood sugar spikes:

FIBRE (veggies) first, PROTEIN second, and FATS and CARBOHYDRATES (starchy grains and sugar) last. Of course, we're not robots – who wants to go around their plate eating in an exact order? However, bearing this in mind can help avoid those pesky blood sugar spikes, and even if you just start eating the first few mouthfuls in this order, it might be enough to make a significant difference.

- Carbs eaten on their own = blood sugar peak and a higher insulin response = louder message to store fat.
- Carbs eaten with protein and fat = lower insulin response = quieter/no message to store fat.
- Carbs eaten after the vegetables and proteins on your plate = quieter/no message to store fat.

Let me explain a few concepts . . .

Eating sugar makes you want to eat more sugar, yet if you skip it for a few days, you lose your cravings quickly – this is simply because you're off the blood sugar roller coaster. In most of these cases, your blood sugar levels will stabilise.

The two main forms of carbohydrate foods are sugar and starches, which are found in foods such as starchy vegetables, fruit, grains, breads, cereals, and rice. I've given some examples already, but there will be more on these foods later on.

Once we eat these carbohydrates, they are broken down into their constituent parts – that is, into glucose molecules, which are absorbed from the small intestine into the bloodstream. Insulin then does its thing, escorting the glucose out of the bloodstream and into the cells.

Our bodies only really like approximately one teaspoon of glucose floating around in the bloodstream at any one time; anything above this must be dealt with by being placed into our cells and stored as energy.

The point is, we want to aim for stable blood sugar levels while avoiding the blood sugar peaks – and the consequent surge in insulin. Blood sugar balance is the gateway to more stable energy, moods and hormones, fewer cravings, and less padding around the middle! If you can get this right, you're more likely to live a longer, healthier life.

> Why you want to avoid dramatic blood sugar spikes
>
> Blood sugar spikes are bad for us because in the short term they can make us feel tired and lethargic – in the long term they can lead to insulin resistance, accelerated ageing, inflammation, weight gain and Type 2 diabetes

Fewer wrinkles, anyone? Too much sugar in the blood also interferes with collagen; it actually causes cross-linking of collagen, which results in our skin stiffening and losing elasticity.

Balancing your blood sugar, and therefore getting your insulin under control, is one of the most important things you can do for your body.

Let's consider these two common examples; we're going to take two pieces of regular, packet-bought, wholemeal bread (as toast), and a medium-sized bowl of pasta to understand their impact on our blood sugar.

	Bowl of pasta Approx. breakdown	2 pieces of toast Approx. breakdown
Total carbohydrates	41.4 g	30 g
Less the fibre	2.4 g	4 g
Net carbohydrates	39 g	26 g

The net carbohydrates that the body converts to blood glucose in the case of the pasta is 39 g (the equivalent of 7.8 teaspoons of sugar), and for the toast, 26g (5.2 teaspoons) of blood sugar – that's a lot of sugar for our bodies to deal with.

You can see that these two examples have lots of carbs and too little fibre – which will cause a blood sugar spike.

That bowl of pasta is going to get broken down quickly due to its lack of fibre; it will have a fast pass through the digestive system. This means it will be digested quickly and the sugar will end up in your bloodstream in no time at all. The pancreas will then move fast and kick out some insulin in its attempt to bring the blood glucose back down to safe levels.

The fibre, on the other hand, doesn't get digested; it just merrily moves down into our colon (the large bowel), where it does lots of good things, such as feeding the good bacteria and keeping things moving. Yes, we're talking regular bowel movements!

High-fibre, good, complex carbohydrates are a much better choice for most of us, as they'll be more filling and are less likely to contribute to weight gain. So, the message here is: eat carbohydrates that have good levels of fibre. I refer to them in this book as **good carbs**, or you may also hear them referred to as **complex carbohydrates.**

You can see why your breakfast of two pieces of toast with marmalade might not be doing you any favours!

Remember: when your insulin level rises and remains high, it's giving your body the message to **store fat, store fat, store fat.** This is because when we have an excess of glucose in the body from eating too many carbs, our bodies can easily convert this sugar to fat.

Additionally, the more frequently your insulin is elevated, the more likely it will result in your cells becoming less sensitive to it (hello insulin resistance and weight gain, especially around the middle). I know, I know, I'm labouring the point – but it's a good point!

I think you get the picture by now: too much insulin is not a good thing! I've talked about it here in the context of weight gain, but elevated insulin is also pro-inflammatory and can increase your risk of heart disease, cancer, diabetes, and strokes.

And, as if that wasn't enough to contend with, you may also find that after eating a carbohydrate-rich meal, your blood sugar crashes. This is because your blood sugar rises sharply – say, after that bowl of pasta – and your insulin production reacts with a similar speed to bring your blood sugar down to safe levels. It often overcompensates, though, which is when you end up with very low blood sugar. Additionally, as your blood sugar plunges rapidly, you'll end up feeling hangry (hungry and angry) – which isn't pleasant for anyone involved!

Some women find that, coming on the back of a blood sugar low, they feel lethargic and irritable – and then hungry again within a couple of hours, at which point the cravings start all over again for... yes, you guessed it, more carbs. It can be a very annoying, addictive cycle. If you find you're hungry every 90 minutes or so, this is possibly the reason.

How To Break The Bad Carbs Habit – And Stop Your Blood Sugar Crashing

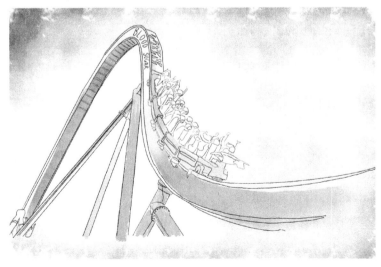

The aim here is to have blood sugar that doesn't peak too quickly and that has a gradual decline over three to five hours. This is what usually happens when you base your diet around two or three wholesome meals a day – which include **the feel-good four** – rather than lots of snacking, or several small meals throughout the day. Your feel-good four meals will fill you up and keep you that way for hours.

You'll be surprised just how good you feel when your blood sugar is balanced! Your mood and energy become more stable and you will lose the cravings for sugary treats, along with the need for constant snacking. It basically puts you back in the driving seat and in control of what you eat.

For most women, it's the too many sweet treats, refined carbs, and constant snacking that lead to weight gain. I see a lot of food diaries where women are doing a great job of eating lots of vegetables and some quality protein, yet when I look closer at the pattern of eating, it's apparent that there are too many snacks in between meals and not enough protein eaten with their main meals. This results in their blood sugar and insulin continuously being spiked throughout the day.

Fat Doesn't Make You Fat

To understand this concept, you need to know that excess sugar gets converted to fat. That's why the adage that 'fat makes you fat' is all wrong – more often, the culprit is sugar! But why? What happens to excess glucose/blood sugar?

Firstly, the body shunts the excess glucose to the liver, forming glycogen (basically, a long chain of glucose molecules, aka stored energy, which is a good thing).

Then, once the **liver-storage depot** is full, the next stop is the **muscle-storage depot**. If you've ever heard of carb loading, this is it: you get your muscles to store lots of energy (glycogen), and then, when you're about to do some endurance exercise, it will keep you going for longer.

So, once the muscle store is full, where to next? The **fat-storage depot**!

Uh oh. And that's why **excess sugar leads to weight gain.**

It's also why you want to avoid eating simple carbohydrates like that big bowl of pasta, or the cake, or the biscuit, or the marmalade on toast – unless, that is, you're trying to gain weight!

Let's look at a scenario of eating a bowl of broccoli.

Broccoli is also a carbohydrate-containing food, but it contains a lot less than the pasta/bread we looked at above.

Let's consider the same size bowl of broccoli (90 g). It looks like this:

Total carbohydrates 6 g

Less the fibre 2.4 g

Net carbohydrates 3.6 g

This equates to less than a teaspoon of glucose that your body must deal with. This means, therefore, less insulin and no message to store fat – which means there isn't any excess glucose for the **fat store**. Plus, it's a highly nutritious food providing good levels of fibre, Vitamins A, C, and K, and lots of essential minerals.

I'm not suggesting that you eat a single bowl of broccoli for lunch, or that you never indulge in a piece of cake or a slice of toast – and, of course, I appreciate that you're probably aware that vegetables are good for you! However, what I'm trying to demonstrate is that, if we ingest too many refined carbohydrates, our bodies break down the sugars quickly, and – over time – this leads to all sorts of health issues, as well as weight gain.

Look around you in most coffee shops and you'll see many people happily consuming croissants, buns, and baguettes (simple carbs that lack fibre) – it's then easy to understand why 60% of us in the UK are overweight or obese. I'm not shaming anyone here. After all, we all know that these types of foods have a great mouth feel and are highly addictive. Nevertheless, I find that once I guide and coach women to see them as occasional treats – and, instead, focus on the good complex carbs as part of the feel-good four – they lose their desire for sweet foods and can get, and stay, on top of their cravings. It can be done!

Remember: simple carbs are broken down quickly by the body, resulting in a surge of blood glucose and insulin. This can lead to insulin resistance and fat around the middle.

We want to avoid a roller coaster-type scenario where we're dealing with peaks and troughs of blood sugar all day long – as well as all the unpleasant side effects and cravings we get after the ride!

If we can't get control of our cravings, we'll never be able to make good choices.

And it's that control that leads to healthier, better choices.

Of course, we're only human and cravings will get the better of us, eventually. That's why no one can stay on a very restrictive diet for long – and why it usually ends up with the yo-yo effect of gaining more weight after losing lots initially.

How Do Slim Women Do It?

If you consider most slim women, they probably don't have an iron will or some superhuman discipline; they're just not that hungry! Therefore, they can say no to cakes and sweet treats – or yes occasionally, depending on their mood. They assert control over their appetite because they're metabolically flexible – meaning they can switch between burning glucose or fat for energy. This is because their bodies handle glucose efficiently and because their insulin hasn't been over-stimulated, which results in freedom from food cravings.

How Can We Achieve This?

At this point, I do, however, want to make it clear that being super skinny is not the point here; it's more about maintaining a weight that suits you, and enjoying a good metabolism that allows your body to function at its best. Society places more value on young, slim women than it does on larger, more shapely, mature women, and that's just thanks to years of crappy patriarchal conditioning. We need more women like Kate Winslet, who are prepared to show their real, beautiful, round bellies and curvaceous figures without feeling the need to change them (see *Mare of Easttown*, where Kate insisted her real body be shown in the intimate shots!) – so that the rest of us feel normal just the way we are.

It's a fact of life that most of us do gain weight at menopause, and if your body is comfortable at a size 14 and you find it impossible to shift the weight, then surely it's better to accept it – whilst still eating healthily and working on your muscle mass.

My aim is to help you achieve a healthy weight that feels good to you! For some women, this means a more curvaceous figure and that's just fine. Look at Nigella! Need I say more?

It's health, happiness, and wellbeing that most of us crave.

ACTIONABLE STEPS

At this stage of our lives, we don't want a diet heavily dependent on simple, refined, beige food, as this will do us no favours whatsoever.

Identifying the type of carbohydrates you're eating – along with limiting the **simple, refined carbohydrates** in your diet – is key. And, if you're going to have something sweet, have it at the end of a meal so it's not going to affect your blood sugar as dramatically!

The good news is, you don't have to avoid simple carbs 100% of the time. Before or after a workout, for instance, they can really have their place – or now and again, when you wish to indulge. It's the ability to get them in the right ratios and to understand the effect they can have on your body that's most important. Then, you can enjoy them as an occasional treat.

Also, bear in mind that some of us deal with carbohydrates better than others. With time, we'll be able to test our bodies to better understand what foods suit us as an individual. However, until then, just listen to your body. If you regularly eat carbs, gain weight easily, and often feel irritable and hungry after a few hours, you may want to reduce your intake. Conversely, if you reduce your carb intake and feel cold and listless, and start to lose weight, you may need to increase them.

This is where **the feel-good four** come in – they will help you feel full and help regulate your appetite.

Did you know that it's now possible to monitor your own blood sugar in real time by wearing a continuous glucose monitor, or CGM? This is a simple device – a sensor that you place on your upper arm, which then translates your blood sugar peaks and troughs into an app, allowing you to see which foods/meals spike your blood sugar and which are better at keeping it more stable. Fortunately, there is no blood involved, like with the traditional methods of monitoring glucose. Personally, I don't think it's necessary to wear it all the time; however, for a month or so it can help guide you as to which foods work best for you as an individual.

Sleep, stress and exercise also affect our blood sugar. Not sleeping well is known to drive your appetite towards higher carbohydrate-rich foods and junk foods the next day. Equally, if you're stressed, this can also drive your blood sugar higher, whereas exercise can help moderate blood sugar; even walking for 10 minutes after a meal can help stabilise blood sugar. So, whilst I have mainly discussed how food affects your blood sugar, and whilst it does have the biggest impact, bear in mind that your sleep, stress, movement, and when you eat also play major roles – more on this later.

CHAPTER 5 ~ FEEL GOOD ABOUT PROTEIN

Now, let's look at **the feel-good four** groups individually, in a little more depth.

Here's the big question: Are you getting enough protein?

Getting enough protein in our diet is essential, now more than ever, because as we age and our oestrogen levels decline, we lose **muscle mass** (known as sarcopenia, which I mentioned before). However, if you wish to go forward with strength and mobility, you'll need to include adequate protein in your diet – on a daily basis – in order to maintain that precious muscle. Additionally, as we grow older we don't absorb protein as efficiently as we did in our 20s and 30s, hence we need to eat more of it.

What else does protein do for us? It:

- turns off hunger hormones
- improves bone health
- helps balance our hormones
- slows down the release of sugars into our bloodstream
- is thermogenic – meaning we burn calories whilst digesting protein as our body creates heat
- is the main component of muscle, bones, skin, hair, nails... in fact, all our cells
- plays a key role in making our hormones, enzymes and immune cells
- gives our body structure
- is needed for brain health and making chemical messengers known as neurotransmitters

Signs you may not be getting enough protein include:

Low stamina/fatigue. Brittle nails Poor skin/hair
Sugar cravings Muscle loss Weak nails
Brittle bones Always hungry Fatigue

Having looked at thousands of women's food diaries, I can tell you that a lot of us are simply not getting enough protein to meet our needs. This is often down to relying too heavily on carbohydrates, or just skipping meals altogether in preference of grabbing a snack.

Protein is essential for us as we go through menopause, not only to stabilise our blood sugar but also to balance our hormones and contribute to our muscles, bones, and overall strength. Let's have a look at where to get it from and how much we need.

Are you familiar with proteins and which foods to get them from? Animal proteins from meat, fish, poultry, eggs, and dairy are like the proteins found in your body. They are complete proteins because they contain all the essential amino acids we need to function, whereas a vegetarian diet – relying on plant protein – may be incomplete because they're missing some of these amino acids. If you're vegetarian, therefore, you need to mix and match and eat a variety of plant proteins over the course of the day to ensure you're getting enough.

Animal proteins include: meat, fish, seafood, poultry, dairy, and eggs.

If you're a vegetarian, you need to think and plan with a bit more vigilance. I find a lot of my vegetarian/vegan clients are lacking in protein and sometimes struggle with weight issues because their diets rely too heavily on carbohydrates. This has a detrimental effect on their blood sugar control and it also means the message to store fat can be louder!

This can, fortunately, be easily remedied – you just need to pay more attention to vegetarian sources of protein (see the table below for guidance). Do also consider your sources of B12 (nutritional yeast is a good source as it can be sprinkled over foods, or take a B12 supplement) and iron, if you're vegetarian or vegan. If you're low in either of these, you'll likely feel tired and lethargic.

> If you suspect you're low in iron, ask your doctor for a blood test before embarking on a course of supplementation – too much iron building up in the body can be detrimental to your health. B12 can be similarly tested. However, this is a water-soluble vitamin, meaning it's generally safer to take than iron as any excess will be lost through your urine.

Personally, I'm leaning more and more towards a vegetarian diet; these days, I find myself eating vegetarian at least 60% of the time (while also ensuring I include adequate amounts of protein). So, why not experiment with vegetarian foods. Your body is a great barometer as to what suits you as an individual, so do pay attention to how foods make you feel once you've eaten them!

Vegetarian sources of B12 and iron (vegans may need to take a supplement):

B12 sources	Iron sources
Dairy products	Green leafy vegetables
Eggs	Eggs
Fortified tofu	Beans, lentils, chickpeas

Fortified milk	Nuts and seeds
Milk	Whole grains
Nutritional yeast	Dried fruit
Cheese	Dark chocolate
	Molasses
	Mussels

Vegetarian proteins include: eggs, cheese, soy like tofu and tempeh, lentils, chickpeas, and beans – although all legumes contain carbs too, albeit the good and complex type.

> Did you know that women who eat more plant-based foods have a lower risk of heart disease and cancer, and may experience fewer menopausal symptoms? Let's consider how to get the balance right.

If you're vegan or vegetarian, I recommend totting up your protein for the day – and do this for a week or so, just until you become familiar with how much you're getting. Then, aim to fill in any gaps if necessary. There are many apps that can assist you, such as MyFitnessPal, MyPlate, and My Macros+. It's a worthwhile investment of your time.

In my experience, women who do increase their protein intake report back that they:

- Are able to curb their cravings more successfully
- Can go longer between meals
- Feel physically stronger
- Notice an improvement in the quality of their skin, hair, and nails.

During perimenopause and menopause, we don't want to lose our precious muscle mass, because this keeps us strong and vital and contributes to a good robust metabolism. Additionally, our bones will lose density as we age, so we want to ensure we're doing all we can to maintain what we already have. Adequate protein, therefore, is essential.

How Much Protein Do You Need?

For women over 40, I would recommend at least 1.1 grams of protein per kilo of body weight – and more if you're doing a lot of exercise.

So, if you weigh 65 kilos, you're ideally looking at:

65 X 1.1 g = 71.5 g of protein per day.

To make it simpler, just aim for 25 g per meal, three times a day – and, if you're someone who works out frequently, increase that to 30 g a meal.

The trick is to get familiar with protein sources that deliver approximately this amount.

Just remember we're all different, and some of us need more protein than others. For example, if you eat 30 g of protein at mealtimes and feel uncomfortable, reduce it a little. However, if you eat 25 g and find you're hungry between meals and always looking for snacks, you know you need to increase the amount – it's a case of listening to the wisdom of your own body.

This way, you're meeting the demands of your own body and responding to your own unique requirements.

Also, know that protein can take anywhere between four to six hours to digest – and it's 'thermogenic,' meaning you use calories/energy to burn/metabolise it.

Bear in mind that when you combine protein with carbs, the carbs don't have a fast pass through your stomach; instead, they must wait their turn to be digested along with the protein. Think of the carbs, protein, fats, and fibre all going into the cement mixer (your stomach) and coming out thoroughly mixed – not a great visual but you get the point! Remember: if you eat your vegetables and protein, followed by the fat and carbohydrates, it can have an even more beneficial effect on your blood sugar levels.

More Control!

Proteins decrease hunger hormones in the brain (such as Neuropeptide Y), as well as reducing the ghrelin we produce – that's the hunger hormone that makes your tummy grumble. Adequate protein eaten at every meal will also increase satiety hormones like CCK, GLP-1, and Neuropeptide Y (NPY), meaning we'll feel fuller for longer and will have more control over what we put in our mouths.

> **Cholecystokinin (CCK)** – a higher amount of these hormones reduce appetite.
>
> We make more of it when we eat protein, as well as fat and fibre.
>
> **Glucagon-Like peptide-1 (GLP-1)** – this decreases your appetite and can help with weight loss.
>
> **Neuropeptide Y (NPY)** – this one stimulates appetite; adequate protein helps keep it in check. High levels of stress can stimulate it, which might explain why some of us turn to food when we're stressed out.

How To Get Enough Protein In Your Meals

How much protein we need is determined by many things, such as:

- How active we are
- How stressed we are
- How old we are.

For now, let's assume we're aiming for 25-30 g of protein. This can look like:

- A three-egg omelette or scrambled egg served with 50g of smoked salmon
- A smoothie with 25g of protein powder / or silken tofu
- A small cup of steel-cut oats (90 g) served with full fat milk/soya milk, 2 tbsp of kefir, and 1 tbsp of toasted pecans
- Half a block of tofu in a stir-fry or curry
- 200g of cooked lentils with an egg and/or 50g of smoked salmon or tinned sardines/smoked mackerel
- 100g of grilled chicken breast
- 100g of steak
- 100g of tuna (no more than once weekly due to the mercury content)
- 100g of white fish
- 100g wild Alaskan salmon

Once combined with other foods such as nuts, seeds, yoghurts, and grains, you can increase the protein content of your meal further.

Protein Sources Guide

Food source	Protein in grams
Set tofu (100 g)	16
Tempeh (100 g)	17

Lentils (100 g raw equivalent to 1 cup cooked 200 g)	18
Chickpeas cooked (164 g/1 cup cooked)	14.5
1 large egg	6
Chicken breast (85 g)	27
Tuna (115 g steak)	22
Salmon fillet (100 g)	24.6
Turkey breast (85 g)	26
Pea protein (20 g) – add to smoothie	20
Whey protein (20 g)	20
Haddock (130 g)	23
Sardines (100 g tin)	23
Oats (1 cup)	11
Milk (1 cup)	8
Yoghurt regular small pot	4
Greek yoghurt small pot	8
Mixed nuts (28 g)	6

This list is just to give you an idea of how to incorporate sufficient protein into your meals. If tofu is your main source of protein, you'll need to eat more of it. As you can see, animal sources of protein generally contain higher levels.

A Quick Reminder On The Importance Of Protein

Protein is an essential part of the feel-good four. It contributes to our health by helping to maintain our muscle and bone mass, and it can help us get on top of our cravings by turning off hunger hormones in the brain and stimulating others that make us feel full. Proteins are literally the building blocks that help us maintain a healthy body.

ACTIONABLE STEPS

1. Eat adequate protein with all meals – use an app to help you.

2. Ensure you have multiple protein sources stocked in your kitchen, such as: cooked chickpeas, lentils and beans (remember, legumes contain both protein and carbs), smoked mackerel, cooked or smoked salmon or trout, tinned sardines (see pâté recipes), boiled eggs, fish, and tofu that can be stir-fried or sautéed and added to a salad. You can also add protein powders or silken tofu to smoothies.

3. If you do snack throughout the day, opt for foods with some protein, such as nuts, seeds, boiled eggs, and nut bites (see recipe).

CHAPTER 6 ~ FEEL GOOD ABOUT CARBS

It's time to upgrade your carbs – and remember: always combine them with proteins, fats, and greens (the feel-good four) to stabilise your blood sugar. Also, eat them last whenever possible.

You should aim to base your choices around:

Legumes, such as lentils, beans, chickpeas and peas
Root vegetables: beetroot, squash, carrots, sweet potatoes, and potatoes with skins
Grains: brown rice, oats (steel cut oats are best), oatcakes, quinoa (technically a seed) buckwheat, millet, sourdough, and rye bread.

And remember: all vegetables and most fruits are good carbs (but don't go overboard – 2/3 pieces of fruit a day and after meals is plenty).

Some Ideas to Get You Started

Instead of toast for breakfast, what about **20-minute oats**?

For this, get a small cup of oats and add a tbsp of flaxseed, a grated apple, and a tbsp of walnuts, and then soak for 20 minutes (the soaking makes it easier to digest). You can then serve with full fat yoghurt, with the oats either heated or at room temperature.

If you like toast, opt for sourdough or rye bread (usually one slice is enough) and top with an avocado. Squeeze over some lemon juice, olive oil, and black pepper, and then add an egg or two – or some smoked salmon or trout to increase your protein. It takes just minutes to assemble and it tastes amazing.

Try a smoothie – see the recipe section.

Try 'legumes for lunch' – and I recommend that we really take this term to heart, as legumes are associated with a healthy menopause. This may be because of their phytoestrogen content (a gentle plant mimicking oestrogen), plus they're high in fibre and very filling.

Use legumes such as cooked chickpeas and lentils as a base for your salads – add rocket, peppers, avocado, and feta, and dress with lemon juice and olive oil. You will then have a tasty and nutritious salad that will keep you full for hours, yet it takes just minutes to put together.

Sweet jacket potatoes are great for lunch, and you can serve them with tuna or beans. Just scrub the skins, rub a little olive oil and salt on them, and place in the oven whole on medium heat for 45 minutes – the prep is much quicker than putting a sandwich together. Alternatively, slice them up, bake them in the oven, and use them instead of bread.

Instead of pasta for dinner, how about a tray of roasted vegetables served with a portion of marinated tofu or fish?

It really doesn't need to be complicated.

Why not use cold potatoes as a base for a salad?

Remember: when you cook and cool potatoes, they make a type of starch called resistant starch – suddenly, the humble potato has more fibre and has become a good and complex carb.

Potato wedges are good too – use organic potatoes and keep the skins on for extra fibre.

Here are some common swaps you may wish to make:

Avoid the simple	Embrace the complex
White/brown bread	Sourdough
	Oatcakes
	Rye bread
Pasta (white)	Red lentil pasta, quinoa, buckwheat
	Chickpea pasta, potato, or sweet potato wedges with skin
White rice	Lentils, chickpeas, beans
	Brown rice, quinoa, millet
Cakes/biscuits	Dark chocolate, walnuts
	Apple and almond nut butter
	Banana and peanut butter

So, remember – when you're eating carbohydrates, your type is:

Good and complex

not simple!

(Maybe just how you like your men, or women!)

Remember: insulin is one of the hormones we do have some control over, so getting it in check is such an important step for your present and future health.

Some Encouragement

Now, let's talk about fibre – it really is a girl's best friend. By eating good complex carbs, we'll also get more fibre into our diet, which is essential in midlife.

Don't underestimate fibre's far-reaching influence on your health! It will help with weight, constipation, energy, immunity, and skin. It's vital!

Guts can become more sluggish in midlife, because oestrogen also affects the motility of the gut. Ensuring we have enough fibre will give our guts a helping hand and keep things moving.

We're aiming for 30 g of fibre daily from vegetables, fruits, whole grains, and legumes (chickpeas, beans, lentils etc.). Here's a good rule of thumb: the more processed the food, the less fibre it will contain.

You can see how easy it is to achieve this in a day by including some of the following foods in your diet. The aim of this list is just to give you some focus, as well as some more examples and ideas of where to find your **fibre** in these **good complex carbs**:

Food	Serving	Fibre in grams
Avocado	half	5
Beans	1 cup	19
Baked beans	1 cup	10
Lentils	1 cup	15.5
Chickpeas	1 cup	10
Chia seeds	25g	11

Flaxseed	1 tbsp	7
Berries	1 cup	8
Broccoli	1 cup	5
Brussels sprouts	1 cup	5
Green peas	1 cup	9
Oats	1 cup	4
Pear with skin	1 medium	6
Apple with skin	1 medium	4
Prunes	6	12
Sweet potato with skin	1 medium	4

According to the World Health Organization, we need between 25-30 g of fibre a day. Sadly, in the UK, only about 10% of us ever achieve this.

How much fibre suits you? If you increase your fibre and find yourself feeling gassier and more bloated, reduce it – we're all very different and require different amounts. I find that some women do well on a lot of fibre whereas others don't need as much. However, it is my experience that, in general, most of us don't get enough.

If you have gut issues, it may be better for you to reduce your fibre / carbohydrates for a while; this will give your gut the chance to rebalance, at which point you can gradually increase them.

What Will All This Fibre Do For Us?

Basically, it will prevent us from overeating, as it will keep us fuller for longer; it stretches the stomach and gives the brain the message that we're full. It literally regulates our hunger hormone, ghrelin, which will consequently prevent overeating.

It will slow down how quickly the sugars from the carbs we consume are absorbed into our bloodstream – hence helping us stay on top of our weight, as well as helping maintain healthy blood sugar control, which is essential!

It can also reduce our risk of experiencing major health issues such as diabetes, heart disease, strokes, and even some cancers.

Fibre provides our gut bacteria (the microbiome – that is, the trillions of microbes found in our gut) with the food they need to grow and flourish. Just think of fibre like a fertiliser for your all-friendly, helpful gut bugs – essential for health.

Fibre helps prevent constipation, and this in turn ensures that we get rid of toxins and hormone metabolites. Constipation can also put extra stress on the liver.

As hormone levels change and our metabolism slows, our guts need a bit more TLC. A sluggish digestion often results in gas, bloating, and constipation.

Fibre is important. It's so important, in fact, that I wanted to give you some background – so that you're enthused and know exactly how to get enough in your diet. You really don't need fancy powders or pseudo foods to achieve optimal levels; it's simpler to just upgrade your carbs.

There are two types of fibre: soluble and insoluble. Think of them like a mop and brush.

Soluble fibre dissolves in water, so you can think of it as a mop – it works by mopping up and absorbing what's in the gut. It can aid in lowering blood sugar (glucose levels) as well as cholesterol levels, and it can soften your stools and prevent constipation.

Find it in foods like blueberries, oats, apples, citrus fruits, nuts, pulses, flaxseed, beans, and lentils…in fact, all legumes. That's why I'm keen to get you eating legumes for lunch!

Insoluble fibre, on the other hand, is like a brush – it tends to help move food matter through the gut, cleaning your digestive tract as it goes. It attracts water, contributes to gut health, and ensures you have regular bowel movements. Additionally, it can help with insulin sensitivity and it can reduce your risk of diabetes.

Find it in foods like leafy green vegetables, root vegetables, carrots, parsnips, potatoes, celery, cucumber, beans, pulses, lentils, nuts and seeds, whole grains, and brown rice.

You can see why we need both for a healthy digestive system.

Don't worry too much whether you're getting soluble or insoluble fibre, as you really don't need to memorise this. Basically, if you follow a whole-foods diet, with plenty of complex carbohydrates – and if you follow the advice and recipes in this book – you'll be eating plenty from both camps.

Fibre And Hormone Balance

Fibre also influences how we metabolise/break down oestrogen. If our gut is sluggish due to a lack of fibre and an imbalance of gut bugs, we may find we're unable to remove and break down oestrogen from our bodies as efficiently as we should, and this can contribute to hormonal imbalances.

Short-chain fatty acids (SCFAs) are also critical for a robust gut – and the gut makes these when there is adequate fibre. These SCFAs not only help the integrity of the gut lining, but they also help with motility and keeping things moving along. They're the main food source for colon cells and have an anti-inflammatory effect.

Fibre, The Great Fertiliser

We really want to think of fibre as a fertiliser for our gut microbes – and it's fibre that encourages the growth and diversity of beneficial bacteria in our guts, which has a profound effect on our health.

We now know that our gut microbes like a good variety of plant-based foods, so keep your vegetables plentiful and varied. One way of doing this is to eat in season – vegetable boxes are an excellent incentive when it comes to variety, especially as most of us are time-poor and prone to buying the same vegetables week in, week out.

Imagine this scenario:

Good, happy bacteria being fed with veg and thriving.

Bad, ugly bacteria (scary spikes) eating sugar/cake and then multiplying.

Remember, we're aiming for 30 g of fibre every day. If you follow these guidelines, you should easily achieve this.

Note: all vegetables have decent amounts of fibre, as do most fruits.

ACTIONABLE STEPS

1. Eat vegetables and protein along with carbs – this slows down the blood sugar response.

2. Try legumes for lunch; get good at the recipes you really enjoy.

3. Stock your cupboard with jars of chickpeas, white beans, packets of red lentils, buckwheat, red lentil pasta, and chickpea pasta.

4. Ensure your carbs include lots of legumes and root and colourful vegetables, and don't rely so much on bread, pasta, and white rice / avoid too much beige! When you do eat these, remember to combine with vegetables and protein – beware the blood sugar spike!

5. Eat fruit after or with a meal, especially if you're watching your weight.

CHAPTER 7 ~ FEEL GOOD ABOUT FATS

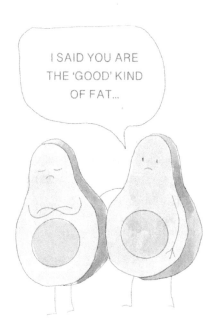

The Headlines

- FATS don't make you fat.
- We need fats to make hormones like oestrogen and testosterone.
- Fats are filling and help curb our cravings.
- Fats turn off hunger hormones.
- Fats carry lots of flavour.
- We need fats to absorb fat-soluble vitamins A, D, E, and K – essential for midlife.
- Essential fats are needed for our joint health and skin.

- The right fats have an anti-inflammatory effect.
- We need fats in order to have a healthy brain and nervous system.

As women start to gain weight, the first thing they often do is cut out fats from their diet – **please don't do this!**

I'll explain why...

If you were brought up in the '70s and '80s, you'll be familiar with the mantra that fat made you fat and would give you a heart attack! Instead, we were encouraged to replace fat with sugar and carbohydrates.

We now know that this advice was unequivocally wrong, but somehow it's had a long-lasting legacy! Excess carbohydrates can easily be converted into fats – a process known as lipogenesis. Lipogenesis is stimulated by a diet that is high in carbohydrates, whereas the process is slowed down when the diet contains adequate fats.

Fats also help us to feel full. When fat reaches our guts, we release a hormone called Cholecystokinin (CCK), which suppresses our appetite, therefore allowing us to hop off the blood sugar roller coaster and take control of our cravings.

That same hormone (CCK) also helps us to feel calm and happy – yes please to that!

Additionally, fat slows down the release of sugars into the bloodstream, helping us dodge the blood sugar peaks we so want to avoid.

Fats carry lots of flavour. For instance, a leafy green salad or some steamed broccoli may seem a bit dull, but if you add a delicious dressing, some good quality olive oil, or some tasty feta, that same salad suddenly becomes a lot more appealing.

Here are some clues that you may be low in fat:

- A Vitamin D deficiency (or a deficiency in other fat-soluble vitamins such as A, E, and K)
- Dry eyes
- Feeling cold
- Dry skin
- Hair loss
- Stiff, painful joints
- Difficulty concentrating/mental fatigue
- Hormonal issues.

A Change in Habits

If we cast our minds back to the 1950s, we can see that women consumed far more fat than we do today, yet their waistlines were considerably slimmer. I believe this may be because they were accustomed to having three meals a day, there was little snacking in between, and meals would have contained unadulterated full fat, which probably resulted in them feeling fuller for longer. My grandmother told me that, as a young woman, she rarely ate outside of the house – unless in a restaurant or on a picnic! I'm sure these habits ultimately resulted in that generation having fewer issues with weight, overeating, and cravings. Additionally, most food eaten away from home is likely to be processed!

Even today, I see women who are fearful of fats – and I get it. After all, that belief has been around for so long, and it's still so ingrained in some people. Besides, we still have athletes on TV telling us that the food they're advertising has the bonus of being low in fat! Unfortunately, low-fat diets often lead to a high-carbohydrate one, which is a contributory factor to weight gain. And that's exactly what happened in the '70s/'80s; fat was demonised, and good honest fats were replaced with too much unhealthy sugar, which in turn contributed to a large swathe of the population getting fatter and sicker.

Why We Need Fats for Hormonal Balance

Women who avoid fats for too long may also end up with a hormone deficiency – not a good idea at this stage of our lives. This is because cholesterol is needed to make hormones; it is the building block for all our steroid hormones, such as oestrogen. Therefore, if we have a dietary deficit, we won't be able to produce adequate hormones. You can see why it's critical that we include fats in our diets.

> 80% of cholesterol is made in the liver and only 20% is influenced by what we eat. Lifestyle factors such as alcohol consumption, a sedentary lifestyle, and a diet high in sugars and refined carbohydrates can negatively affect our levels. In other words, dietary cholesterol from fat gets a bad rap, but the reality is, dietary cholesterol has little influence on our levels and is not the whole story when it comes to elevated cholesterol.

As you can see from the diagram below, in order to make oestrogen (as well as other steroid hormones like progesterone, testosterone, etc.) a women's body must go through several steps – and the first one is having adequate cholesterol.

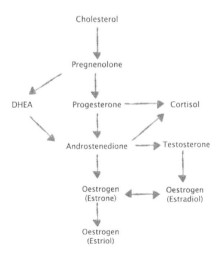

Hence, in order to support your hormonal health, you need to eat a diet with adequate amounts of fat.

The Benefits of Fat Continued...

As fats help us to absorb our fat-soluble vitamins such as vitamins A, D, E, and K, they are critical for immunity, vision, bones, hair, skin, and healthy ageing.

As fat doesn't break down into glucose like carbohydrates, it doesn't have the same impact on our blood sugar curve – and it doesn't require insulin.

Fat will also keep you fuller for longer; it's estimated that fat takes several hours to transit through your stomach and small intestine, helping you get on top of those incessant cravings.

Fats To Avoid

The only fats that should be totally avoided are... **man-made ones.**

Avoid Hydrogenated Fat/Trans Fat

Basically, this is a fat that has been altered to behave differently, like sunflower oil becoming a margarine – and, therefore, hard at room temperature, when its natural state is fluid. It is basically a pseudo fat, and evidence shows that this kind of fat is the most damaging to your health. Back in the '70s and '80s, we were eating lots of margarine instead of good old butter – a more natural food that we've been eating for centuries. These days, manufacturers use safer methods to produce margarines, and these types of fats are being phased out of baked goods etc., but you get my point – stick to the natural stuff!

These days, the kinds of fats you really need to avoid are those that have been used at very high temperatures and used to cook with repeatedly (think processed foods like crisps); these can produce damaging compounds, and they're not good for human health.

Instead, you can cook mostly with olive oil, as it has so many brilliant properties. Other oils you might want to cook with include, rapeseed oil, avocado oil, and – occasionally – butter and coconut oil (which are higher in saturated fats but have other valuable properties).

> My top 3 fats to cook with are extra virgin olive oil, coconut butter and butter – tried and tasted foods that been around for a long time. For dressings, I use olive oil, walnut oil and avocado oil. Whilst seed oils are not inherently bad for us, many of us consume too many of these, which can cause an imbalance and inflammation in the body.

Most seed and nut oils are generally better enjoyed at room temperature, such as in a dressing.

We're only human, and who doesn't like a few crisps now and again? But do keep these foods to an absolute minimum and think of them as an occasional treat. If you stick to whole, real, unprocessed foods most of the time, you won't have a problem.

Saturated Fats

These fats, which are hard at room temperature, include animal fats (such as the fat in beef or the crispy skin of chicken), butter, and cheese. They're also found in foods like sausages, cakes, biscuits, chorizo, salami, and bacon.

These types of fats have been associated with health risks, especially heart disease (and remember: women after menopause have a much greater risk of heart disease).

Remember: foods like cheese and yoghurt are minimally processed, so choose full fat and really savour them. For most of us, there is little evidence that they are detrimental to our health or our cholesterol levels.

Whilst we don't want our diets to be heavily dependent on foods like butter, cheese, and red meat – because they may have an inflammatory effect on our bodies and may raise our LDL cholesterol (the bad type) – at the same time, they shouldn't be demonised. There is no evidence that saturated fats in their entirety are inherently bad for us. Some people may be able to eat a lot more without risk, whilst others do well to eat less, depending on their genetic make-up. At this moment in time, I believe it's better to err on the side of caution until we can easily test for these genetic differences.

How much is too much? Current recommendations are that no more than 10% of your daily calories should come from saturated fat – but, like I said, it is highly individual. For most of us, this looks like 20g/ 4 teaspoons of saturated fat a day.

Fats To Focus On

Dr Mark Hyman talks about getting an 'oil change' by replacing the bad fats with good fats, which is a great way to think about it. These are the ones you want to focus on...

Monounsaturated And Polyunsaturated Fats

These fats are liquid at room temperature, and – as they're associated with many health benefits – they are where we should be looking for most of our fat consumption. They're also associated with lowering our risk of heart disease.

However, you will see seed oils in a lot of processed foods – eaten like this, they're not so good! Remember: keep all processed foods to a minimum.

These fats include olive oil, nuts and seeds, avocados, olives, and oily fish.

Extra Virgin Olive Oil

This oil is an absolute must-have in midlife because it contains plant compounds called polyphenols. Polyphenols are plant chemicals that can lower your risk of cancer and cardiovascular disease (because they help keep your blood vessels flexible and healthy), protect your brain, improve your immunity, and slow down the ageing process. Their effects are far-reaching, which is probably one of the reasons why the Mediterranean diet remains one of the healthiest diets on the planet.

Aim for 2/3 tablespoons daily.

Omega-3 Essential Fatty Acids

These are found in oily fish – such as salmon, sardines, and mackerel – as well as in flaxseed and walnuts. In my experience, most people are not eating enough of this type of fat.

We also want to ensure these long-chain fatty acids show up in our diet on a regular basis, as they can really help us through and beyond midlife; they can help reduce symptoms associated with menopause (such as joint pain and depression), lower the risk of osteoporosis, contribute to vaginal health, reduce inflammation, and protect our hearts and brains.

If you're not eating oily fish a couple of times a week, think about taking a good quality fish oil – or, if you're vegan, an algae oil supplement. And remember: they're called essential for a reason!

How To Include Enough Fats In Your Meals

Here's a list of the fats that I feel offer us the most benefits:

- Extra virgin olive oil – for salads and dressings, drizzled over food, and used in shallow frying. Use olives as a pre-dinner snack.
- Wild or sustainably farmed oily fish, such as salmon, trout from chalk streams, sardines, herring, and small halibut.
- Flaxseed or flaxseed oil (not heated).
- Nuts/nut butter, and seeds and their oils (generally not heated).
- Avocado or avocado oil – OK to heat. This oil contains lots of Vitamin E and biotin, which your skin and hair will benefit from too.
- Coconut oil – for cooking stir-fries and curries, or for baking (yes, it's a saturated fat, but it's a medium-chain fatty acid, which just means it's more likely to be used for energy). It also rich in lauric and caprylic acid which have antibacterial / antifungal properties.

How much FAT should you eat?

Aim for a total fat intake of 25-35% of your daily calories with no more than 10% coming from saturated fats. Of course, there will be days when you have more or less, and it will be highly dependent on you as an individual. This advice is a rough guide because, in the real world, very few of us have time or need to calculate our macronutrients on a daily basis – and we all have a unique set of circumstances and unique bodies. Therefore, always listen to your body, and pay attention to how you feel.

Confused about serving sizes? Here's a rough guide for everyday life:

FATS AND OILS	SERVING SIZE per meal
Extra virgin olive oil	1 tbsp
Coconut oil	1 tbsp
Pumpkin seed oil	1 tbsp
Avocado	half an avocado
Butter	2 tsp
Avocado oil	1 tbsp
Olives	4-6
Nut butter	1 tbsp
Nuts	25 g or a third of a cup
Eggs	2/3

ACTIONABLE STEPS

1. Cook with **olive oil** as much as possible (it has a four-thousand-year track record and is minimally processed). Alternatively, use **coconut oil** and occasionally **butter**.

Oils like rapeseed, soya, and avocado are also suitable for high-temperature cooking.

2. Try adding a good quality extra virgin olive oil to your meals as a condiment like Mediterranean people do; they literally pour it over their food. Invest in a good one – see it as a supplement, because it is positively contributing to your health.

3. Ensure that all your meals contain some fats – this could be olive oil, eggs, avocado, fatty fish like salmon, sardines (regularly), cheese, olive, nuts, chia, flaxseed, tahini, or nut butters. Remember: including fats in your diet is going to fill you up, meaning you won't be tempted by sugary snacks.

4. When making supper, enjoy a few olives whilst cooking and avoid that bowl of crisps.

CHAPTER 8 ~ FEEL GOOD ABOUT GREENS

Greens can help with:

- weight maintenance
- ageing well
- healthy bones
- disease prevention
- ensuring we get enough vitamins, minerals, phytonutrients, and antioxidants in our diet
- aiding with detoxifying hormones and chemicals from the body
- heart health.

Greens are brilliantly helpful in midlife; they're significant contributors to our health and therefore deserve a generous allocation on our plates.

They include the following (and the ones in italics are cruciferous too – more on that below):

Beet greens, bok choy, broccoli, Brussels sprouts, cabbage, chard, collard greens, courgette, *cress,* dandelion greens, green beans, iceberg/romaine lettuce, *kale,* micro greens, mustard greens, peas, parsley, rainbow chard, *rocket,* romaine lettuce, spinach, Swiss chard, turnip greens, *watercress,* and small leafy greens like coriander, parsley, mint, sage, and thyme.

Basically, anything green (as long as it's edible)!

Greens Are A Powerhouse Of Nutrients

Greens are packed full of vitamins such as A, C, E, and K, and – as well as folate – they also contain iron, calcium, and an array of antioxidants. Greens are high in fibre, and they contain an array of polyphenols. These disease-fighting compounds, which help these same plants survive in nature, seem to exert a similarly protective effect on us, shielding us against disease.

Bone Health

Bones are constantly breaking down and building back up again, but when oestrogen is in low supply, the building-up part slows down – therefore, it's a good idea to focus on what we can do to minimise bone loss. See the chapter on better bones for more info. on how to take care of yours.

The **calcium**, **magnesium,** and **Vitamin K** found in greens are key components of strong, healthy bones. One small study showed that women who ate one cup of greens daily lowered their risk of hip fractures by a whopping 45%.

It's not quite as simple as this, as there are many other factors that contribute to strong healthy bones – such as our oestrogen levels, our alcohol intake, how much and what type of exercise we do, and our stress levels. However, including greens in our diet is a significant step in the right direction.

Greens Aid Our Natural Detox Systems

Alcohol, medications, pollution, pesticides, chemicals, heavy metals, and plastics all find their way into our bodies through what we eat, breathe, and place on our skin. We're detoxing these 24/7 – this process never stops, not for birthdays, not for Christmas, and certainly not for that big night out. Our bodies just keep on keeping on. Eating greens regularly can help our bodies deal with this onslaught.

Heart And Cardiovascular Health

Women have a lower risk of heart disease compared to men – that is, until they reach menopause and lose the protective effect of oestrogen. One way oestrogen protects us against heart disease is by helping us produce a gas called nitric oxide. This gas is an essential aid when it comes to the widening of our blood vessels while also retaining their flexibility – this, in turn, can help prevent high blood pressure, strokes, and heart disease! The good news is that you can eat dietary nitrates, which can also help you to produce nitric oxide and to enjoy the same benefits.

Greens with a good nitrate content include: Swiss chard, celery, lettuce, kale, spinach, cabbage, and rocket.

Don't worry about focusing on just these ones; I've listed a few to give you an idea of where to find them, but in general, any dark green leafy vegetables are a great source.

> BEETROOTS are also an excellent source of nitrates, even though they're not green. Do check out the recipes for beetroot, aim to eat it a few times a week, and enjoy the benefits!

Variety Is Key

It's worth remembering that we're aiming for a variety of vegetables, so don't just opt for spinach every day and nothing else. Sometimes, it's easy to fall into the trap of thinking that a little bit of something is good for us, so a lot might be even better – but this is often not the case! **Variety, variety, variety** – that's where it's at. A weekly vegetable box is a great way to max out on nutrients.

Spinach contains **oxalates,** which can bind up calcium and prevent your bones from absorbing it – so you can see why eating it every day might not be a good idea.

Instead, enjoy it just a few times a week, and use a variety of other greens such as kale, mustard greens, watercress, romaine lettuce, broccoli, lamb's lettuce, etc.

Brain Health

Studies show that just 1 cup of dark green leafy vegetables may help protect us from cognitive decline and memory issues. So, you should aim to make this a habit – remember to keep a green drawer or box in the fridge, as this way you'll always have some to hand.

Cruciferous Vegetables – Another Bestie

Broccoli, Brussels sprouts, cabbage, cauliflower, Romanesco cauliflower, collard greens, kale, and rocket are some great examples that contain powerful compounds called sulforaphanes and indole-3-carbinols.

These substances can help with the liver's detoxification processes, enabling the body to neutralise toxins, reduce inflammation, and protect our DNA more efficiently. They can also upregulate functions in the liver that help us detoxify oestrogen safely, which may lower our risk of breast cancer. Breast cancer is a complex disease, of course, but hey, why not do everything you can to put the odds in your favour?

Once we've used our oestrogen, it needs to be cleared by the body. Some oestrogen metabolites – that is, the by-products of oestrogen breakdown – can go on to damage our DNA if not cleared efficiently from the body.

Broccoli is one of the hardest hitters when it comes to these compounds.

It's worth putting some effort into getting to know how to make these vegetables zing, and then work them into your diet so that they're regularly showing up on your plate.

ACTIONABLE STEPS

1. Aim to have a green salad daily. If you can get into the habit of having a salad as a starter this will also help your blood sugar control.

2. Lightly sauté kale, chard, or spinach and add to an omelette.

3. Blend a handful of greens into a smoothie.

4. Throw a few handfuls of greens into a soup, casserole, chilli, or pasta sauce – the perfect way to enjoy them in autumn and winter.

5. Make a kale pesto and use it as a condiment.

6. Keep some frozen broccoli, spinach and other greens in your freezer so you always have some to hand.

7. Try the broccoli recipe in this book and get into the habit of having some pre-cooked greens sitting in the fridge (top shelf), ready to go. For a great addition to a salad or as a side, add a little lemon juice and some tahini – delicious!

8. Remember to have a dedicated drawer or area in your fridge where you always have some greens to hand. Aim for a variety of local produce if possible as it's usually so much higher in nutrients.

It needn't be complicated – it's simply a case of grabbing a handful of rocket, or steaming/sautéing some greens with your meals. You won't believe the difference in how you look and feel when you start adding greens to your diet on a regular basis.

There are no guarantees in life when it comes to health, but I view greens as a little extra health insurance.

Check out the recipe section for two of my favourite dressings to enjoy with your greens and salads!

TIP: Even just a bit of olive oil and balsamic vinegar can make greens so much more appealing.

CHAPTER 9 ~ FEEL GOOD ABOUT TIMINGS

When To Eat – Tune Into Your Midlife Body Clock

Hopefully, you now understand how to incorporate the basics of **the feel-good four** into your meals and, therefore, how to have an overarching structure to your diet.

Now we need to focus on WHEN to eat the feel-good four.

Timing Is Everything

"If your eyes are open, your mouth doesn't need to be" – Satchin Panda.

> Now, more than ever, is a great time to get in tune with yourself – because, in midlife, we want to give ourselves every advantage going forward. When we eat, some would argue, is just as important as what we eat; it certainly has a major impact on our health.

First, I would like to draw your attention to the benefits you can experience by eating in tune with your body clock.

Have you heard of the term 'circadian rhythm'? It refers to our natural, daily rhythm – our internal clock, if you like – that regulates our sleep-wake cycle. It repeats every day and is governed by the amount of light and dark we're exposed to.

Our bodies are so influenced by this day and night cycle that so many things – including our hormone production, how hungry we are, how well we digest and convert food to energy, our sensitivity to insulin, our temperature control, how we feel psychologically, the quality of our sleep, and our risk of chronic diseases – are all affected by it!

According to Doctor Satchin Panda (a leading expert in the field of diurnal/daily eating, and professor at The Salk Institute, an acclaimed scientific research centre in the US), by eating in an 8-12-hour window we are giving our bodies every advantage in maintaining our health.

Every single cell in our body has a biological clock that responds to light and darkness. When we disrupt this natural cycle with a late night, looking at our screens until bedtime, or even being inside all day and not exposing ourselves to enough daylight, our body gets confused and isn't able to follow this essential rhythm.

> Screens emit a blue light that tricks our brain into thinking it's still day. Cells in the retina are activated to produce a photopigment called melanopsin in the presence of blue light, which in turn decreases our melatonin (our sleep-aiding hormone), and... boom! We have disrupted sleep – especially the deep, restorative kind, which we need now more than ever!

If we eat little in the morning and then have most of our calories when it's dark, we can also confuse our body clocks. Our bodies are naturally primed for food earlier in the day, when we're more sensitive to insulin. That's why it's never a good idea to eat and drink late into the night – late-night calories aren't treated the same way and can lead to health issues and weight gain.

I find that a lot of busy women skip breakfast, and then tend to eat more calories at the end of the day. When you're perimenopausal and your hormones are on that roller coaster, the body needs as much stability as possible.

Why Get In Tune?

Eating in tune with our body encourages more restorative sleep, and that deeper sleep literally helps our brain rid itself of toxins. This is why poor sleep is associated with many diseases, especially dementia and Alzheimer's, in later life.

> Cognitive decline is much higher in women than in men. In fact, your chance of getting Alzheimer's is 2:1 if you're a woman post-menopause!

By being exposed to bright light in the morning, we help set our circadian rhythm, while dim light at night helps us build melatonin (the hormone that helps maintain our sleep cycle).

Overnight fasting for 12-14 hours gives our bodies the opportunity to repair and rejuvenate.

Additionally, leaving a three-hour gap before bed (when you don't eat) will also improve sleep quality, as well as help with fat burning overnight – meaning you'll feel fresher the next morning.

A good night's sleep also helps with weight maintenance – insulin becomes more sensitive when we follow this pattern, hence we have better blood sugar control, which results in more control over our appetite and fewer cravings. Have you ever experienced the ravenous appetite that follows a bad night's sleep?

I think of fasting as a 'fine-tune' for our bodies.

What can we do to tune ourselves up and enjoy all the health benefits that come with eating in time with our body clocks?

During my decade of working with women, I've found that this pattern works wonders for weight loss/weight maintenance and wellbeing, especially as we transition through peri-menopause and adjust to post-menopause.

A Word About Fasting

There is no doubt that fasting is inherently good and natural for us as human beings. I have found that, for most midlife women – who wish to enjoy the benefits of fasting but at the same time need to work it around their busy lives, their energy requirements, and fitting it in with their families – the following patterns work wonders and are the most sustainable.

Firstly, aim for an eating window of 10-12 hours.

TIMINGS

This is a guide – choose the timings that work best for you and your life.

Breakfast	Lunch	Dinner	Snacks
8–9 am	1–2 pm	6 –8 pm	Mid-morning or late afternoon. Skip the snack if wanting to lose weight!

The aim is to maintain a gap of four to five hours between meals – the time it takes for the food to pass through your stomach and into your intestine. If you do this, you'll also get a mini-fast and be primed for fat burning. If you eat your feel-good four, you'll easily achieve this gap between meals.

With time, you'll get into sync with this rhythm and your appetite will adjust until you're not hungry every couple of hours! It will also give you a rest from constantly digesting food.

After all, the gut needs time off too – for a bit of housekeeping and cleaning up – and it's the job of the migrating motor complex, also known as an 'interdigestive housekeeper', to step in when you stop eating. Think of it like this: you can't clean up the kitchen while the party is in full flow... so give that gut a rest.

> A lot of us are accustomed to snacking throughout the day – because our meals haven't been filling enough and didn't include the feel-good four, or because it's just a habit we've become used to. Have a think about what your pattern looks like and ask yourself if it's making you feel good.

Three meals a day and one snack work well for most.

If you're trying to lose weight, you may want to skip the snack, but let's be realistic – most of us like a snack or a mid-morning coffee.

So, why not aim for the following?

A 12-hour gap overnight – between dinner and breakfast.

Aim to stop eating around 7/8 pm so you can enjoy an overnight fast of at least 12 hours. If you can extend it to a 13/14-hour fast, even better.

After 8 pm, you could decide that your kitchen is CLOSED!

Water, black tea and coffee or herbal teas are OK, but if you're adding milk or sugar, it doesn't count towards your fast.

Changing your own timings can be difficult to start with. However, as with most things in life, it's just a case of:

PRIORITISE LATER OVER NOW – the benefits will be well worth it.

> Most of us are better able to deal with carbohydrates in the morning when our insulin maybe more sensitive. Have you noticed that, in the evening, it can be tricky to feel full? I know I have in the past; I just wanted to keep eating. However, if you follow this pattern, your body will simply adjust to it in time.

Most of us are just little habit machines! With effort, determination, and know-how, however, we can replace unhelpful habits with healthier ones – and never look back!

If you do find yourself feeling hungry after your evening meal, just know that – with time – your eating patterns will adjust. Just because it's tricky for the first week or so, it doesn't mean it will continue to be so hard once you've established the pattern. And remember: this lovely overnight gap means you will wake up hungry, your digestive juices will be flowing, and you'll really enjoy your breakfast or brunch. With time, your body will adjust to these timings, and soon it will become no effort at all.

Also, bear in mind that your body is more likely to store calories eaten later in the evening as fat rather than burning them for energy, which can lead to weight gain. It can also result in feeling hungrier the next day and slowing down our metabolic rate, meaning we'll burn fewer calories.

If struggling with late-night munching, distract yourself – phone a friend, get out of the kitchen, go for a walk... anything that appeals, really. Say to yourself, "I'll be eating again tomorrow, what's the urgency?" We can find treats in other areas of our lives – it doesn't have to be food-related – and usually, within 30 minutes to an hour, your craving will pass anyway.

Not Hungry For Breakfast?

Many clients tell me they're never hungry for breakfast, but when I question them as to what time they stopped eating the night before, they'll tell me they had a snack at 10 pm. You may find you're hungrier for breakfast if you've had a sufficient overnight fast. Remember: your digestive system needs a break – plus, when you eat late into the evening, you're also switching off your precious overnight fat burning.

However, breakfast isn't for everyone, and if you want to fast until lunchtime and you feel good doing that, go ahead – it might work better for you, but don't do it just so you can snack late at night.

Always adapt timings and advice to your own needs, so it makes you feel good. We're all unique and by the time we're in our 40s and 50s, we know our bodies well – trust in yours when choosing what pattern suits you best.

I call this the **Take Control Three Meals A Day Plan:**

Breakfast	Lunch	Dinner	Snacks
7 – 8 am	12 – 1 pm	6 – 7 pm	Mid-morning or late afternoon

3 meals a day

1 snack if necessary/coffee

4/5-hour gaps between meals/for at least one meal

Nothing except water in between, or teas/coffees without milk and sugar

All eaten within a 12-hour window e.g. 7 am to 7 pm.

Alternatively, try this:

The Hybrid Eating Structure

Brunch	Snack	Dinner
10 – 11 am	4 pm	7 – 8 pm

This is for just three or four days a week, eating in a 10-hour window, hence fasting for 14 hours. It involves a large brunch at 10 or 11 am, and then a meal at 7/8 pm, with a snack if necessary in between.

Then you can return to the Take Control Three Meals A Day eating pattern (three meals a day in a 12-hour window) for the rest of the week.

> As I write this, I'm having a little giggle to myself! It's not exactly groundbreaking advice to eat three meals a day, but so many of us don't have any kind of structure around our eating patterns, falling into the trap of snacking and imbibing milky drinks all day long – I'm talking lattes and flat whites (and yes, they contain a type of sugar... lactose). However, if you can work on your own timings and instil a structure around your diet, you'll find you'll be back in the driving seat and, consequently, back in control of what and when you eat.

Perhaps try to alternate between the two structures dependent on the demands and energy requirements of your day. This has worked wonders for some women who wish to lose weight, as well as those looking to have more energy and clarity; they report feeling fresher, lighter, and more in control of what passes their lips. Others prefer to stick with the three meals a day and an occasional snack, and feel more balanced following that structure.

Why not experiment with it and see what works for you?

> The average person eats in a time window of 15 hours :(
> Give a woman a break!

Of course, there will be days when life just gets in the way – you may have social events you wish to join in with, you may not observe the four or five-hour gaps, you may get tempted by an extra snack or even miss the 12-hour eating window altogether... but really, don't worry. Just know that if you can maintain this solid foundation for your diet – even for five days a week – I'm confident that you will notice the benefits, such as sustained energy, better mood, and weight maintenance. It's so worth the effort of getting this right!

> **The Importance Of Light**
>
> It is equally important to aim for some time outside each and every morning, even if just for a few minutes. This morning light can help our internal clocks set themselves up for the day; not only is this helpful in influencing our diets, but it also positively impacts our mental health.
>
> **Light is measured in lux**

> **OUTSIDE, you're exposed to 10-20,000 lux**
>
> **INSIDE, it's just 200-800 lux**
>
> Idea – why not have your first cup of tea outside, take some calls whilst walking, and reply to your messages? Just get out as much as you can.

Troubleshooting The Transition

You don't need to be afraid of hunger. You may feel hungry in the four to five-hour gaps initially, but it will pass.

Bear in mind that a lot of us are used to the feeling of being full but considering how feeling lighter in our stomach is an equally lovely sensation, why not embrace it?

Hunger won't hurt you. Whilst you don't want to get to the point where you're about to keel over, feeling hungry two hours after a meal doesn't necessarily mean you urgently need to eat or that you're in any kind of danger! Why not give your body a chance to burn its stored sugar and fat for energy, if needed? You'll find that, as your blood sugar control improves, you'll experience fewer hunger pangs.

I appreciate this can be tough when we live in a world where sugary cheap processed food is so readily available, but it's just a case of doing your best. YOU CAN DO THIS!

What if you're still hungry after finishing a meal? Well, the 20-minute rule comes in handy here; after this time, the craving usually passes as our brain picks up the message that we've had enough food.

> Eating your meals slowly helps, so try putting your cutlery down between mouthfuls, and always be the last to finish at the table. You'll feel fuller sooner and your digestion will thank you too!

We eat for many different reasons, so it's good to recall this simple acronym when you have the desire to keep eating after a meal. Just ask yourself: Am I feeling any of the following...?

H. Hungry?

A. Angry?

L. Lonely?

T. Tired?

Of course, there are lots of reasons why we overeat, which is why it's a good idea to work with a coach or psychologist if you're finding it hard to control. This can also really help in terms of uncovering what drives your overeating. However, if you can't do that, just talking things over with a trusted friend can be very useful. Of course, they can't offer professional advice, but they can listen – and sometimes, the reality of saying these things out loud can give you a better understanding of yourself. This alone can be a great start.

It's also a good idea to have meals at regular times, as you'll feel the benefits of eating in tune with your circadian rhythms.

I've suggested timings here, but this is just a guideline – make it your own and change the timings to ones that suit you best.

If you do just one thing after reading this chapter, then make sure you get that 12-hour overnight fast.

Most perimenopausal and menopausal women are more concerned with losing weight, but if you're someone who has suffered from – or currently has – an eating disorder, I would emphatically encourage you to seek individual help with your approach to your midlife diet.

Please note: if you're diabetic or have a health condition that adversely affects your blood sugar, then seek the advice of a health professional before embarking on any kind of fasting. Generally, however, fasting is beneficial.

Final Thoughts

By observing these timings:

- you're going to be in better shape
- you're going to become a more efficient fat burner
- you're going to have fewer cravings
- you're going to reduce your risk of diabetes
- you're going to feel more energised
- you're going to sleep better
- your digestion will improve
- your mood will be more stable
- you'll be ageing gracefully
- you'll decrease your risk of getting all the most common diseases
- you'll feel good in menopause.

Dr Satchin Panda advises us to set clear deadlines:

My kitchen closes at _____ (?)

My light turns off at _____ (?)

Aim to be consistent, but don't get disheartened if it's tough to begin with. I find that, initially, it's just a case of getting over the unwillingness to change habits – then, once you experience the benefits, you'll be much more inclined to stick with them.

I call it 'pushing through the pain barrier' and 'getting into a growth mindset', and it can often take five days or so until your body adjusts to these new habits and timings. Remember: it's just a temporary discomfort! Also, if you're hormonally challenged (what most of us refer to as feeling hormonal) and want to snaffle up all the chocolate in sight, you'll find that this approach will dampen that effect... eventually!

If you're interested in Dr Satchin Panda's fascinating work, do look at his website, where you can participate in his ongoing studies – you can find information on the app, myCircadianClock, plus lots of interesting lectures on YouTube. He's also written the book, *The Circadian Code: Lose Weight, Supercharge Your Energy And Sleep Well Every Night*.

I've just referred to Dr Satchin's work here, however, there is a lot of research to support the hypothesis that fasting is inherently good for the health of human beings. But, as ever, you're in the driving seat – experiment and see what works for you.

CHAPTER 10 ~ FEEL GOOD ABOUT WHEAT

A Word About Wheat – Do You Need To Be Gluten-Free?

(Full disclosure: I'm not wild about wheat, especially the heavily processed kind!)

In my experience I find a lot of women are too dependent on wheat – and I believe it contributes to weight gain and other health issues when eaten in excess. As I've said before is 60% of the population is either overweight or obese. Could there be a link? I'm not saying that wheat is the only culprit here – it's certainly the culmination of lots of sugary, processed foods – it just happens to be that wheat is the grain we most commonly consume.

I was certainly my biggest and unhealthiest self when I ate toast for breakfast, sandwiches for lunch, and pasta for dinner – plus, I frequently suffered from indigestion and bloating. When I first began practising nutrition, I was reticent to encourage the removal of wheat from my clients' diets, but now – having seen lots of food diaries over the years, and observed the corresponding person sitting in front of me – I've concluded that, for most of us, too much wheat (of the processed kind) is not doing us any favours.

There are many reasons why people struggle with wheat – especially bread – but, generally, if you have a wheat allergy (rare) or coeliac disease, you'll know you can't have any at all. However, if you suspect you react to eating wheat, have a nutrient or an iron deficiency, or suffer from osteoporosis, it would be worth getting yourself a coeliac test to rule it out.

Coeliac disease is a serious condition that affects the lining of the gut; it affects the body's ability to absorb nutrients, hence minerals like iron and calcium can become depleted. It affects approx. 1 in 100 people. If you're concerned, raise your issues with your GP, who can easily screen for coeliac by running a simple blood test. Some people don't get diagnosed until they're in their 40s and 50s.

Most women I work with report feeling fine when eating wheat some of the time, but at other times they suffer from bloating, fatigue, diarrhoea, and headaches. Due to this inconsistency, they don't contribute these symptoms to wheat. However, I have observed that when they remove or dramatically cut down their wheat intake, these same clients report their symptoms disappearing altogether.

In midlife, our guts can become more sensitive and sluggish due to hormonal shifts, and this can result in a weakening of our digestive power. For some, the hard-to-digest food is wheat, in its many forms – such as packet bread (brown or white), pastries, cakes, biscuits, and flour. I'm sure that, by now, you're identifying these as simple carbs so you're aiming to cut back on them anyway :)

Modern Bread Isn't That Great!

Have you noticed that bread lasts so much longer these days? You can have it in a cupboard and still be eating it five days later – it still feels squishy and fresh. Well, this is due to the undesirable enzymes added to the flour, and it certainly isn't the bread our parents or grandparents were brought up on.

In 1961, a method to make bread known as the Chorleywood process was invented. This process required additives and more yeast to make the bread rise faster – unfortunately for us, it meant we were eating a highly processed foodstuff with little nutritional value. Additionally, wheat has been hybridised to produce higher yields – great for feeding the world, maybe, but not so great for our guts!

Consider this: if you make bread at home, all that's required is flour, yeast, salt, sugar, and butter – that's just five ingredients. Compare that to shop-bought bread and you're looking at 15-20 ingredients at least (check out the labels), including preservatives, enzymes, emulsifiers, and flour treatment agents. These can do a real number on our gut and microbiome – that is, our collective gut bugs, which play such a vital role in keeping us healthy.

Watch out for **flour treatment agents** – basically, chlorine and chlorine dioxide... yuk! There is much controversy in the scientific community regarding the safety of these agents. However, manufacturers continue to use them.

Trace amounts of these chemicals probably won't do you any harm – that is, if you're only eating them now and again. If you ingest them day in, day out, year in, year out, however, then you may be asking for trouble!

What About The Gluten?

Gluten is a group of proteins found in wheat, rye, spelt, and barley. It's what helps the bread rise. When flour is mixed with water, these gluten proteins form a sticky, glue-like property that traps the carbon dioxide, which is why bread rises and has a springy, chewy texture – and which is why it's so delicious and addictive! Gluten, in fact, comes from the Latin word for 'glue'.

Generally, it's wheat that tends to cause most issues, whereas rye, barley and spelt? Not so much – probably due to their less processed nature.

However, no human can fully break down that sticky, gluey protein, and this is why it's an issue for some.

Now, there are a few underlying issues that you might want to think about...

The Most Common Issues With Wheat

Many women who are intolerant to wheat suffer from bloating and cramps, most likely because their gut bacteria start fermenting the undigested gluten, and then... boom! They have a pregnant belly of air! Not a pleasant experience.

Others may be reacting to the additives, preservatives, and yeast in bread; too much yeast in the gut can result in discomfort and bloating.

Another reason people suffer after eating wheat is because it contains a fermentable carbohydrate known as a FODMAP food.

What are **FODMAPS** (fermentable, oligos, di-, monosaccharides and polyols)? These are carbohydrate foods that are poorly absorbed in the gut, and that are prone to absorbing water and fermenting in the colon. They're notorious for triggering digestive symptoms in people with IBS. You find them in many foods but, **for most of us, they're not a problem**. If you suffer from IBS, a low FODMAP diet is often recommended for a SHORT period of time; it's never meant to be a long-term diet.

Weight Gain?

In my experience, women who rely heavily on bread and pasta tend to struggle more with their weight. This is simply because these foods can be broken down into simple sugars very quickly and, therefore, spike your blood sugar levels. I'm picking on wheat as it is most ubiquitous, but any processed food can have this effect.

However, avoiding bread for a period, and working on your gut health, may alleviate these issues – often resulting in a more tolerant gut.

Avoiding Wheat For A Couple Of Weeks

Why not give wheat a miss for two weeks and see how you feel – see if it's worth the sacrifice of giving it up for a while? If it's beneficial to your health, and if your gut is more comfortable, the sacrifice might be worthwhile. You can then return to it, and you may find that you can tolerate it much better. You may also come to the realisation that eating bread in the morning is OK, but if you eat it at night, you don't seem to tolerate it as well.

Most of my clients report that their guts feel more comfortable once they reduce their wheat intake. Plus, eating less wheat can help you eliminate processed food – which is a GOOD thing and will really benefit your overall health.

Wheat is everywhere – and we eat so much more of it these days – but as a plant, it has radically changed over the years. Today, there is a new fast-growing variant with a greater gluten content that requires more pesticides! Bread is also made in a less traditional fashion, which affects its digestibility.

Takeaway

If you suffer with the symptoms discussed above, why not give wheat a wide berth for a few weeks to a few months and see how you feel?

My approach with many of my clients who have gut symptoms like gas, bloating, and general discomfort, is to take wheat out of their diet for a month or so. If there's no underlying issue, they can often reintroduce it into their diet in smaller amounts without any adverse effects.

If you feel like you have no issue with wheat, I would still recommend having it no more than once a day. You really want to avoid the toast for breakfast, sandwich for lunch, and pasta for dinner scenario – it may be troubling even the most robust gut and crowding out health-giving foods like legumes and vegetables.

If you continue to enjoy wheat, why not switch to the more traditional foods, like sourdough, and buy organic (not sprayed) where possible?

Sourdough Is A Much Healthier Choice

Proper sourdough contains just three ingredients (flour, water, and salt), and it's made over 24 hours using traditional methods and a live starter that contains a beneficial bacteria called lactobacillus.

Because sourdough is fermented for hours, the gluten is broken down and becomes more water-soluble – hence it is easier for you to digest.

Gluten-Free Alternatives?

Also, don't be tempted to replace bread with ultra-processed gluten-free alternatives; it's the carbs, glucose, and blood sugar roller coaster we're trying to take you off. Good carbs, remember?

I don't want to demonise bread – you should still enjoy the odd toastie, croissant, birthday cake etc. now and again (I do)

– but try to avoid becoming too reliant on it. In most cases, your body will thank you.

Takeaway

Most wheat:

- is highly processed
- is heavily sprayed with pesticides
- contains FODMAPs and yeasts, which may be a problem for some
- converts to sugar easily, and therefore may lead to weight gain.

ACTIONABLE STEPS

Aim for natural, naturally gluten-free alternatives.

Legumes (such as chickpeas, beans, and lentils), rice, quinoa, buckwheat, millet, potatoes, and sweet potatoes – these are all great bases for salads and soups.

Choose more traditional forms of bread.

Instead of eating bread, why not slice up some sweet potatoes and bake in the oven for 20 minutes with some olive oil? Check out the sweet potato bread brunch in the recipes section.

Learn to love sourdough.

Choose sourdough and rye bread over processed packet breads.

Have just one slice of bread at a time instead of several.

CHAPTER 11 ~ FEEL GOOD ABOUT ALCOHOL

Are you someone who turns to wine for a bit of a pick-me-up, or for something to look forward to at the end of the day? A bit of solace, a habit you've got into? I know many of us do, and while – initially – it can help you feel more relaxed and cheerful, this effect is short-lived and does us no favours in the long run.

Most of us like a drink here and there, and let's face it – it's an incredibly sociable thing to do. Besides, just the ritual of making a G&T or anticipating an elegant glass of rosé can feel like such a treat.

However, it can be all too easy to get into the habit of overconsuming, as well as getting used to that initial hit of the feel-good neurotransmitter, dopamine.

FYI

Progesterone declines from perimenopause, which results in lower levels of GABA (gamma-aminobutyric acid).

GABA promotes calmness, good mood, and sleep – so with little or no GABA, it's no wonder that some women turn to alcohol to get the same effects.

Exercise, magnesium, green tea, and a whole-foods diet can also improve your levels of GABA.

You may have noticed that you just don't tolerate alcohol as well anymore, and that hangovers, red faces, and waking up hot in the middle of the night – and no, not that kind of hot! ;) – are much more likely. Regular drinking to numb menopausal symptoms is not helpful ;(.

Is It Worth It?

Excess alcohol can increase our risk of breast cancer, osteoporosis, and future health issues, as well as exacerbate other symptoms associated with menopause.

What's A Woman To Do?

Whilst I'm not suggesting you become teetotal, I do think it's a good idea to understand how alcohol affects you, and how to approach – and enjoy it – in the healthiest way possible!

Why can't we tolerate alcohol as well anymore? What changes in midlife?

1. The alcohol we consume is more concentrated in the body.

Compared to our younger selves, we have a lot less fluid in our bodies to dilute the alcohol. This effect also happens to men to some degree – at last, a bit of equality! ;)

2. We make less of the enzyme that's required to break it down.

This enzyme, alcohol dehydrogenase – try saying that after a few drinks! – helps us process alcohol. With less of this around, the alcohol hangs around in our bodies for longer and we feel its effects more acutely.

3. Our livers may also be a little slower in metabolising generally – add alcohol to the mix and your poor liver can become overwhelmed.

Why It's A Good Idea To Drink Less

Alcohol inhibits our deep sleep cycles, and usually results in us waking in the middle of the night (and missing out on that health-giving restorative sleep). Even if you feel like you get off to sleep more easily after a few drinks, the net effect is less quality sleep.

> Good sleep is so vital to our health, and prioritising it in midlife is essential.
>
> TIP: Why not have your glass of wine at lunchtime, or early evening, and give yourself more time to process it before bed?

Alcohol can result in dilated blood vessels, which may trigger/exacerbate hot flushes in some women. So, if you suffer from excessive heat, it might be worth having a break from alcohol for a week or two to see if it helps.

Alcohol also depletes our B vitamins – which are essential for hormone balance, energy, and our nervous system – and low levels of these B vitamins can increase anxiety and irritability.

Alcohol changes the way oestrogen is broken down in the body, as well as increasing the levels of circulating oestrogen by up to 10%. That's one of the reasons it's a risk factor for breast cancer. Some of us are more at risk than others – for example, having dense breasts and/or a family history of breast cancer. However, according to Cancer Research UK, only 5-10% of breast cancers are due to an inherited faulty gene; most are down to diet and lifestyle.

If you're taking HRT, you'll want to reassess your approach to alcohol – because both HRT and alcohol are independent risk factors for breast cancer.

Excessive alcohol is also incredibly ageing.

Too much alcohol can lead to weight gain; most people think this is because of the sugar content, however, most alcoholic beverages contain very little sugar, the sugar in drinks is often down to what's been added, like fruit juices in cocktails. The reason that alcohol can cause weight gain has more to do with how our body is processing it; the detox process becomes a high priority, and the processing of other nutrients (such as fat, protein, or carbs) is delayed. It literally slows down your fat burning – not a good idea! Alcohol is also calorie dense: it has 7 calories per gram as opposed to 4 calories per gram for carbohydrates and protein.

Alcohol may contribute to unstable blood sugar levels, which can result in cravings! This is because some alcoholic drinks (cocktails or drinks with fruit juice) cause a rapid peak in blood sugar. We've all been there: a couple of glasses of fizz or a cocktail on an empty stomach and, suddenly, you're ravenous – at which point the well-intentioned healthy eating you were planning goes out the window.

Excessive alcohol is also bad news for bones – too much alcohol can increase your risk of osteoporosis.

Too much alcohol does a number on our gut too. The good bacteria can literally be sloughed away when we consume alcohol (consider how we use alcohol to sterilise things – do we really want to do that to our guts?). Alcohol also affects the integrity of the gut lining, which is important for our overall health and may lead to intestinal permeability (leaky gut - this is when our guts lose their integrity and bacteria and toxins can pass through the gut lining and into our bloodstream – not a good idea!).

Alcohol depletes many vitamins and minerals.

It's also incredibly dehydrating. Wrinkly skin, anyone?

Alcohol is converted by the liver to a metabolite called acetaldehyde. This compound is very toxic and is often the culprit behind hot flushes, headaches, nausea, and a racing heart. The body eventually breaks this down into carbon dioxide and water – it's key, therefore, that we detox efficiently so that this toxic compound doesn't hang around too long!

What Is Moderate Drinking Then?

The UK's Chief Medical Officer recommends that both men and women consume no more than 14 units per week, which is about six glasses (175 ml per glass) of wine. I don't understand why there's no differentiation here between men and women – we're smaller, as are our livers, plus we have more body fat that retains alcohol, so surely it follows that alcohol will be more concentrated and have a more dramatic effect on a woman's body! So, bear that in mind when you're considering your 14 units per week – or when trying to keep up with a male partner.

That's enough of the bad news… let's look at the good news!

For some of us, enjoying a nice glass of something can be very enjoyable and is a major part of our culture. I know from experience that bonding over a few drinks with other human beings can be incredibly good for the soul – and bonding is vitally important for our overall health. Therefore, my aim here is to give you the knowledge and motivation so you can make your own mind up as to how much, and when, you choose to drink.

Some studies even demonstrate that moderate drinking may have specific health benefits. Moderate drinkers tend to have a better bone profile, decreased risk of cardiovascular issues, and a lower risk of stroke – although, as far as breast cancer is concerned, any amount of alcohol can increase your risk, albeit small!

What is moderation? The studies quote anything from one to two drinks per day – and, of course, there are many other factors to consider, such as your size and how fast you as an individual deal with the alcohol.

Of course, there could be other factors at play. Moderate drinkers, for instance, may also be more likely to be moderate in other areas of their life: they may eat less, consume more nutritious foods, exercise regularly etc., so this might have a bearing on these beneficial results.

So, how can we enjoy a drink and still feel fantastic?

Firstly, I think it's important to become aware of how much you're drinking, and to take control by keeping tabs on it.

Secondly, listen to your body. If you're someone who drinks a glass or two of wine and suffers from a hot flush (some do, some don't), wakes up in the middle of night, or feels hungover or suffers from headaches the following day, that's a bit of a clue that you're not dealing with alcohol very well and that you need to rethink your approach to drinking.

Advice For A Balanced Approach To Drinking

If you still wish to enjoy a drink but want to remain healthy, as well as looking and feeling amazing, here's how:

1. Never drink on an empty stomach. Either nibble on some nuts, olive, or cheese beforehand, or better still, enjoy your favourite tipple with meals – this basically slows down the absorption rate of the alcohol and it may also enhance the

liver's ability to clear it. Therefore, it doesn't have such a negative impact.

2. Use a smaller glass – choose one that feels a bit special.

3. Invest in a spirit measure, then measure out your drinks: e.g. 25 ml for spirits (1 unit) and 125 ml for wine with 12% ABV (1.5 units). Most wine is served at 175 ml (2.1 units). I know it sounds over the top, but just do it until you're au fait with measures – your body will thank you!

4. Drink the best stuff you can afford, and sip s l o w l y. Really savour it. The average woman can break down approximately one alcoholic drink per hour, so go slow.

5. **Aim to have three to four days off a week – this is crucial.**

6. Keep a diary and record how much you drink – seeing it in black and white really helps.

7. Try an app – the MyDrinkaware app can record your units for you.

8. Enjoy your drink earlier in the day and avoid alcohol in the three hours before bed.

I find that once clients are coached on how to approach alcohol in a more healthful way, they report back that they can now tolerate it more – without the negative side effects.

What To Drink On Your Nights Off?

On my nights off drinking, I tend to make myself something special – like tonic water with grapefruit or lime, a sprig of rosemary, and lots of ice. Preparing a lovely, appealing drink for yourself is a nice ritual to get into whilst cooking dinner or winding down at the end of the day.

A **pomegranate** juice with ice also makes for a nice drink, and it's a great way to enjoy this fruit's powerhouse of nutrients. I don't usually recommend drinking juice – due to its effects on your blood sugar – however, I can make an exception here. Additionally, pomegranate encourages the growth of a bacterium in the gut called Akkermansia – and individuals with good levels of this bacterium tend to be healthier and live longer. Plus, remember: the polyphenols help look after our cardiovascular system.

Why not drink it from a nice wine glass, add some ice, and dilute 50:50 with sparkling water or tonic? It's delicious and still feels like a treat!

A word of caution: if you're trying to lose weight or are diabetic, it may be better to drink it with your meal to prevent a blood sugar spike.

You can also drink **coconut water kefir**, which contains beneficial bugs. Be aware, though, that you should start low and slow; too much good bacteria all at once can overwhelm the unprepared gut.

There are also lots of **alcohol-free beer, wine, and gin alternatives** that are getting better all the time. However, watch out for the sugar content with these!

Or how about trying one of the two following non-alcoholic drinks? They've proved to be very popular amongst my clients – and me :)

Kombucha – a fermented fizzy tea that tastes a little sweet and a little tart; it's a good replacement for sparkling wine.

REAL Kombucha is a fabulous brand that I've served at dinner parties, and that friends thought was alcoholic fizz. It's light and incredibly subtle. See the resources at the end of this chapter – Royal Flush is my favourite and has proved to be popular.

Wild Eve is another firm favourite – it's a delicious, delicate-tasting botanical infusion that contains adaptogens that may help you feel more relaxed. It's made by a talented herbalist on the Isle of Harris from the herbs and flowers grown there.

Use it like a spirit and blend it with tonic or sparkling water. A 25 ml shot contains a mere 20 calories! Although, the best thing about it is definitely the taste. The downsides? It's a bit more on the expensive side and, sadly, a bottle doesn't last long – but only because everyone loves it!

What About Alcoholic Drinks? The Low-down

What does a drink look like in terms of units?

175 ml glass of wine = equivalent to 2.1 units

(although, often, pubs serve 250 ml – that's 3 units!)

A gin and tonic – 1 shot (25 ml) = 1 unit

A glass of Champagne – 125 ml = 1.5 units

A beer – one pint = 2.3 units

So, you can see how easy it is to exceed the recommended maximum of 14 units per week!

Best To Worst

Clear spirits such as **vodka, gin, and tequila** contain no additives or sugar and are therefore processed more quickly by the body. Incidentally, if you have one shot (25 ml), this is equivalent to only 1 unit of alcohol – compare that to a small glass of wine (175 ml), which contains 2.1 units. Drink your G&T with a low-sugar tonic water, plus lots of ice, and you'll find it lasts a lot longer too.

Light beers have fewer calories, and even normal beer only has 4-6% ABV (alcohol by volume), so it's also a less alcoholic choice than wine or spirits – as long as you don't drink copious amounts!

Champagne tends to have very strict regulations and high standards, resulting in lower levels of mould toxins compared to those found in some beers and wine. A small flute (125 ml) of Brut Champagne is also lower in calories (80-100 calories).

Red wine is touted for its polyphenol content, a powerful antioxidant that is associated with preventing heart disease and that may improve blood flow, as well as contributing to better levels of HDL – the good cholesterol.

If you look at the Mediterranean diet, which includes moderate amounts of red wine, then it seems it has a good track record.

Red wine is actually believed to be one of the most beneficial alcoholic drinks due to its high levels of polyphenols. This is because, in the process of making red wine, the red grape skin encounters the liquid for a lot longer than it does when white wine is being made. During this fermentation process, the polyphenols are converted to over one hundred different polyphenol chemicals that will not only benefit the gut, but also the cardiovascular system and your overall metabolism. Therefore, it may be beneficial to swap your white or rose for red.

Whisky, brandy, bourbon – these 'darker drinks' are said to be hangover-inducing because they contain congeners, which are harder for the liver to clear (although there is no clear evidence for this).

Remember to enjoy the best wine you can afford and have it with a meal. Additionally, try using smaller glasses and sipping more slowly, or opting for clear spirits like gin or vodka.

> Why not serve your drink of choice in a beautiful glass? And take half a glass at a time; it will really help to slow you down and you won't feel like you're missing out. Also, don't forget to use a shot measure to ensure you're not exceeding your units.

The Benefits

We can spend a lot of time and money on gym memberships, fancy face creams, facials, and make-up with the aim of looking and feeling better, yet we often overlook the most obvious culprits that are robbing us of our looks, our energy, and our health.

This certainly applies to alcohol, especially when too much is consumed. It can leave us both looking and feeling tired and dehydrated, and it can also lead to weight gain and depression; just what we don't need when we're going through menopause.

The great news is, just cutting back for a short period of time can really show up in your appearance and wellbeing. My clients tell me that when they cut back, they feel brighter, enjoy a more stable mood, have higher energy levels, generally feel more up than down, have less brain fog, have clearer eyes and more radiant skin, and are less prone to weight gain and hot flushes. Who doesn't want that?! It's worth the sacrifice when you look at it like this.

Some of the women I work with tell me they drink because of the social pressure put on them to do so, rather than any real desire of their own... but remember: **saying YES to others may be saying NO to yourself!**

If you enjoy alcohol, drink it on YOUR terms.

ACTIONABLE STEPS

How about doing these three things to help you achieve a better balance with alcohol?

- **One** – Try 14 days without alcohol and then get into the routine of four alcohol-free nights a week.
- **Two** – Take a photo of yourself right now, and then take another in four weeks' time, after you've cut back on the alcohol. Visual proof is such a good motivator. You may be surprised by how much your appearance changes after just a few weeks of cutting back (or complete abstinence).
- **Three** – On your nights off, experiment with your own non-alcoholic beverages until you find something you really enjoy and look forward to. It's hard to start with, but so very worthwhile.

I've really laboured the point here, but that's because cutting back on alcohol – if you're prone to overconsuming – is going to have a massive impact in terms of making you healthier... probably more so than just dietary changes alone!

> TIP: Read this chapter again when you feel you need more motivation.

Resources

REAL Kombucha
https://realkombucha.co.uk

Wild Eve
https://www.wild-eve.com/shop/p/wild-eve-botanical-infusion-recipe-no-1

CHAPTER 12 ~ FEEL GOOD ABOUT STRESS

Cultivate Calm And Control Your Cortisol

In this chapter, let's talk about **stress** and its effect on **cortisol** – how does it impact us in midlife?

We've covered how we can influence insulin, now let's consider cortisol; as I've mentioned, it's the other hormone we can assert some control over. Let's look at why it's so important at this point in our lives.

As our oestrogen and progesterone hormones start to fluctuate, and ultimately decline due to our ovaries shutting up shop, our body must adapt to this lack of sex hormones. This is where the adrenal glands step up to supplement us with small amounts of oestrogen and progesterone. However, our adrenal glands are also responsible for producing cortisol, a bossy little hormone that will take over, given half the chance. When we experience stress, the body will always choose survival over reproduction and, therefore, the adrenal glands focus their efforts on making cortisol at the expense of other hormones – specifically progesterone. We then end up being out of balance. Sadly, if this happens too frequently, our emotional and physical wellbeing really takes a hit.

What Is Cortisol?

Cortisol is a vital hormone that is key in terms of how our bodies respond to stress. It regulates our blood pressure and our insulin, it helps convert food to energy, and it reduces inflammation. The problem begins when we produce too much for too long – in other words, when we experience chronic stress.

Signs that your cortisol is too high:

- Waking up in the middle of the night
- Sleep issues
- Weight gain
- Thinning hair
- Blood sugar issues
- Dry mouth
- Headaches
- Loss of libido
- Mood swings
- Anxiety and depression
- Digestive issues
- Getting sick often
- Heart palpitations
- Over or undereating.

You can see why it's imperative that we keep our cortisol levels in check. So, let's learn how to do just that!

What It Does

We produce cortisol when we sense danger. Basically, our brain sends a message to our all-important adrenal glands (two little almond-sized glands that sit on top of the kidneys) to release two hormones: adrenaline initially, and then, to maintain the stress response, cortisol. What follows is an increase in blood pressure, heart rate, and blood sugar. The flip side of all this action is that anything your body doesn't consider to be urgent – such as your digestion, your repair mechanisms, and your sex drive – are all dialled down. This makes absolute sense: in the short-term, prioritise survival.

However, this evolutionary response, which is vital, was only ever designed to be a temporary state.

When cortisol floods our system, it's difficult to think straight, especially if you find yourself in a negative situation. Long-term stress has a negative impact on our brain too; it literally shrinks the hippocampus.

I'm sure you don't need me to tell you that, in modern life, more often than not, the stresses we encounter are rarely dangerous or physical; they're more likely to be emotional or social. Let's face it – not many of us need to run away from a sabre-toothed tiger or put up a fight against the local alpha female from a rival village (as much as you may feel like it when you're having a menopausal meltdown).

The kind of stress we experience is more likely to stem from an overwhelming to-do list, a sick family member, a demanding job, stroppy teenagers, poor health, money worries, and so on.

Why is chronically elevated cortisol such an issue for midlife women?

It's an issue because…

1. Cortisol will instruct your body to pump some of your stored blood sugar into the bloodstream, which sounds like a good thing – you'll be burning more calories, right? Wrong! Because, most of the time, whatever is stressing us out doesn't require any physical action! Chronically elevated cortisol can often lead to weight gain, especially around the middle – evolution puts it here so that the body can access it quickly.

Unfortunately, weight gain is all too common in women who are chronically stressed. Of course, you could counteract this by sprinting off into the distance every time you feel stressed out ;)

2. Secondly, recall that we're less resilient and more prone to getting stressed because there is less oestrogen and progesterone available; our female hormones do a great job of buffering stress. Hence, if we're stressed during perimenopause and menopause, it's a double whammy! The adrenal glands are doing their best to produce our sex hormones – however, they just can't do this if survival is the priority.

3. Thirdly, high cortisol has a negative impact on our thyroid and may result in low thyroid function. This can result in a slower metabolism, weight gain, and feeling cold and tired. Elevated cortisol can also block or lower the production of our other sex hormones – oestrogen, progesterone, and testosterone. Like I said, it's a bossy little hormone that can really take over!

4. Fourthly, our digestion, absorption, and immunity will take a back seat if we're stressed out. Cortisol curbs functions that are non-urgent and, over time, this may result in digestive issues and getting sick more often!

You can see why it's imperative, now more than ever, that we pay attention to our stress levels and aim to mitigate stress the best we can.

Whilst too much cortisol is associated with stress and negative effects on the body – such as weight gain and lowered immunity – it's worth bearing in mind that, like most things in life, it's all about a healthy balance.

So, how do we get our cortisol to follow a healthy daily curve? For example, peaking in the morning (to get us up and out of bed), and then gradually declining throughout the day, so we're nice and sleepy by bedtime?

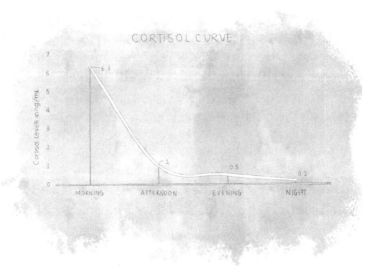

Figure: CORTISOL CURVE — Cortisol Levels in ng/mL plotted against MORNING, AFTERNOON, EVENING, NIGHT. Values shown: 6.3, 1, 0.5, 0.2.

What Can We Do To Bring Our Cortisol Back Into Balance?

So, what can we do in the moment, when anxiety or stress kicks in?

How about trying one of these breathing techniques?

1. Take the index finger of your left hand and run it over the little finger of your right hand. As it traces up from the base to the top, BREATHE IN, and as it traces down the other side, BREATHE OUT. Continue this action over the rest of the fingers and the thumb. This act of breathing – along with the physical sensation of touching your fingers – is very effective at lowering your stress response. Just one round helps, but two or three are even better.

2. When feeling anxious, STOP, take a few deep breaths, and identify where you're feeling the stress in your body. Bear in mind that most of us breathe shallowly, especially when we're stressed or anxious, so interrupting this with slow, deeper breaths can be really beneficial. We often hold tension in our bodies – common areas where this tension can build up are our shoulders, necks, jaws, and pelvic area. Wherever you hold yours, focus on that area as you breathe in and out, slowly, through the nose. While doing so, visualise letting go of that tension. This simple act can be very calming to your mind and body, and can highlight exactly where your body is tensing up.

3. Try the 4-7-8 breathing pattern known as 'Relaxing Breath', as recommended by Dr Andrew Weil. He describes it as a natural tranquilliser for the nervous system and recommends it to all his patients.

Not only is it a great technique to use in the moment to calm you down, but it can also have cumulative effects if practised regularly.

How To Do It

Slowly breathe in through the nostrils, with your mouth closed, to the count of 4.

Hold to the count of 7.

Exhale through the mouth, making a whooshing sound, to the count of 8.

Do this for four rounds, twice daily.

Why not tag it onto a daily habit, such as after brushing your teeth or before eating breakfast and lunch? Whatever works for you.

Long-term – To Keep Your Calm Vibes Going

1. Practice 10 minutes of meditation or mindfulness. This can just be 10 minutes per day, either using an app like Calm or Headspace for a guided experience, or just sitting comfortably somewhere and observing your breath.

For some, meditation means just getting comfortable with your thoughts – if you can't sit down and do this for 10 minutes, then it's probably an indication that you're overly stressed. Of course, not everyone wants to sit; you might find you can get into the same calm observational state by walking in nature or swimming. Do what works for you, but do make it a daily practice.

These days, there's so much evidence showing that mindfulness can support brain function (remember, it's essential as we age) and keep our cortisol levels in check.

2. Forest bathing – also known as shinrin-yoku – is the habit of spending time in forests, which has been popularised by the Japanese. It's been shown that getting out in nature can lower cortisol levels. One study even revealed that a daily, one-hour walk in nature was more effective than taking an antidepressant!

Find a green area and see it as your sanctuary.

> Did you know that trees give off volatile organic compounds called phytoncides? When we walk in forested areas, we breathe in these plant chemicals, which can have a positive impact on our immune system and increase our ability to fight off infection.

3. Let go of perfection. Sometimes, a 7 out of 10 is good enough.

4. **Get outside in the morning**. This simple action and exposure to more blue light can help set our daily rhythm and contribute to better sleep.

5. View some of your stresses – such as those that have meaning in your life – as positive things, rather than seeing them as insurmountable or as situations that threaten you. Research shows that your response to stress is much healthier if you can view stressful situations as challenges that you're capable of overcoming. If you can respond with this kind of control, you will feel better initially, as well as feeling healthier in the long-term.

> According to Kelly McGonigal (a leading health psychologist and inspiring lecturer at Stanford University), how you respond to stress matters to your brain and your body. She says, **"Go after what creates meaning in your life and then trust yourself to handle the stress that follows."** Your body responds to this in a much healthier way.

6. **Recognise how you respond to stress**. Are you a fighter, a flighter or a freezer? I used to be a fighter, and my goodness has that got me into some trouble and altercations over the years! Instead, recognise which you are and ask yourself: is that reaction really serving YOU?

7. **Catch it early**. One of the most effective ways to control your stress response is to recognise when it's happening. By using a calming technique, such as breathwork, you can stop yourself from spiralling out of control or relying on sugary treats and alcohol as a coping mechanism.

Of course, all of this requires being self-aware and looking at yourself objectively (not an easy task, I know!); this is where mindfulness and meditation can give you an edge, and the ability to view yourself from a distance.

8. Exercise – when I joked about going for a run every time you feel the stress response surging through your body... actually, it's not such a bad idea, just not very practical for most of us! You could, however, do some squats or at least move your body in some way. Research shows that exercise can help bring your cortisol levels back into balance. And, of course, being active throughout the week will also help your overall cortisol rhythm. Aim to move your body for at least 30-60 minutes every day.

However, too much exercise can have the opposite effect. Many endurance athletes have elevated cortisol, so running a marathon every other day isn't where it's at – for most of us, at least! Also, if you're very tired and are pushing through a gruelling workout, it can often make matters worse.

9. **Laugh!** Laughter is the enemy of cortisol – it calms the stress response and helps us produce serotonin, dopamine, endorphins, and oxytocin. I've also heard laughter being described as the shortest distance between two people – bonding with others is another great way to feel calm.

10. And, finally, you have to evaluate your daily life: are you saying yes to others and no to yourself? Are you rushing around and being unrealistic about how much you can fit into your day? If so, remind yourself that life is short and to be enjoyed. As women, we have been juggling our kids, running a home, our careers, our parents etc. for decades. Menopause is the perfect time to reflect if this is at the expense of our own well-being and ask ourselves: is it time to redress the balance?

Cortisol And Our Diets

Balanced blood sugar can very much contribute to healthy cortisol levels too, and when we're stressed we burn up a lot more nutrients, so be sure to follow the feel-good four and avoid processed food as much as you can.

We can also deplete our magnesium, B vitamins, and Vitamin C when under stress, so you may want to focus on these if you feel you've experienced chronic stress recently.

Magnesium-rich foods include:

Pumpkin seeds, almonds, dark green leafy vegetables, dark chocolate, avocado, oats, legumes – don't forget 'legumes for lunch' – and whole grains such as brown rice, millet, oats, buckwheat, and rye.

Foods that are rich in B vitamins:

Legumes, dark green leafy vegetables, meat, poultry, fish, whole grains, eggs, dairy, nuts, and seeds.

Foods that are rich in Vitamin C:

Kiwis, oranges, blackcurrants, peppers, broccoli, and herbs like thyme and parsley.

You're probably thinking that, by now, I've covered most food types, and you'd be right; if you eat real food, and digest and absorb it well, you'll be covered. For a lot of us – especially when stressed – we don't eat as well, or digest our food as thoroughly. This is where supplements can come in handy.

Supplements That Can Help During A Stressful Period

Like with all things, it's never just one thing; I find a lot of women take a cocktail of supplements in the hope that it's a one-way ticket to reducing stress. It isn't!

However, there is evidence supporting the effectiveness of the following two supplements, and I find they make the biggest difference to women.

Magnesium – when we're stressed out, we use up far more of this all-important mineral and can end up with a deficiency. Low levels of magnesium in the body mean we don't cope with stress as well, resulting in more cortisol. Plus, a magnesium deficiency is also associated with reduced levels of serotonin – which is a mediator for anxiety.

Why not try a therapeutic dose of 300-400 mg daily, divided between two doses, such as a capsule with breakfast and one with dinner?

If taking any medication, always check with a healthcare professional that it is suitable to take alongside a supplement.

Ashwagandha – this is an ancient medicinal herb that has been used for 3000 years to relieve stress. It may be helpful in helping to normalise cortisol levels, hence reducing the stress response.

Try 250 mg once or twice daily.

I find that some women swear by ashwagandha, whereas others don't notice much of an effect. If you're feeling stressed, why not try it for a month and see if it helps? I recommend using it for short periods whilst you're bringing your body back into balance.

Epsom Salt Baths

Why not treat yourself to an Epsom salt bath? There's a lot of anecdotal evidence to show that it can relieve stress and anxiety. It can also help relieve muscle tension, which is especially important in the shoulders, neck, and spine if you spend a lot of time in front of screens. Most people report feeling more relaxed after an Epsom salt bath, and it can be a nice relaxing habit to get into before going to bed. Why not try it a few nights a week?

You can use 300 mg of Epsom salts dissolved in a bath, and even soaking for just 15 minutes is enough time to reap the benefits. If you have any type of skin inflammation or infections, however, then this isn't recommended.

CHAPTER 13 ~ FEEL GOOD ABOUT YOUR GUT

Your gut microbiome: the healthier it is, the healthier you will be.

The microbiome is just the term given to our collective, individual gut bugs (which are as individual to us as our fingerprints) – that is, the trillions of micro-organisms that live in our gut and have a major influence on our bodies. They outnumber our cells by 10 to 1, so it's no surprise they have a major influence on our physical and mental health – especially as there are roughly 1000 different species! Basically put, these gut microbes play an **essential** role in how healthy we are.

Having a healthy gut microbiome is essential when navigating through menopause, because microbes in the gut influence how we break down and metabolise hormones. If this process isn't happening efficiently, it can lead to an imbalance and inflammation. Oestrogen and progesterone receptors are found throughout the gut, hence during perimenopause and menopause, we can experience more gut issues. However, if your gut bugs are in good shape, you are less likely to have as many menopausal symptoms. So, with that in mind, let's try and make them as healthy as possible!

A good, diverse microbiome also has a major impact on our immunity; it's estimated that 70-80% of our immune cells reside in the lining of the gut.

Where Bacteria And Immune Cells Hang Out

70% of immune cells are located just outside the lining of the gut, whereas our gut bugs (the microbiome) are located on the inside lining of the gut – they're separated by a wafer-thin lining, allowing them to communicate easily. This is why the health of your gut has such an impact on your immunity.

Our gut bugs also influence our weight and our mental health.

How To Take Care Of Yours!

To maintain your gut bugs – as well as keeping them happy and plentiful – you'll need to take care of them on a daily basis.

You've probably heard about probiotics and prebiotics, and may be wondering what the difference is.

Probiotics contain live bacteria – they add live organisms to your gut – and they are found in foods like live yoghurt, kefir, sauerkraut, miso, kimchi, and kombucha. They can also be taken as a supplement.

Prebiotics are foods that contain non-digestible fibre-like vegetables, fruit, and legumes, and they can help the growth and diversity of your gut bugs. Some examples of foods that contain these include bananas, Jerusalem artichokes, onions, garlic, leeks, and oats.

Whilst probiotic supplements have their place for some individuals – say, after a course of antibiotics or for an individual with specific gut issues – a healthy diet from a variety of plant-based foods is going to make the biggest difference and supply you with the diversity of bacteria and yeasts you need to thrive.

What The Gut Microbes Don't Like

- Stress – it interferes with our digestion and our delicate balance of gut bugs. Adrenaline can literally encourage the growth of the less desirable, unfriendly gut bugs!
- Alcohol – traditionally, we used alcohol to sterilise things. It can have the same effect on our gut bugs too!
- Late-night eating has been shown to detrimentally affect the microbiome and cause an imbalance. Plus, recall how the body is more likely to store late-night calories as fat instead of burning those calories for energy – so don't forget to have that 12-14 hour fast overnight!
- Preservatives and emulsifiers – which are found in most processed foods – also have a detrimental effect on our little critters.
- If you're a fan of artificial sweeteners, you may want to think again, as they may stimulate appetite and contribute to weight gain and obesity – the very things they're supposed to be protecting you from! Sweeteners also have a detrimental effect on your gut bugs. If you really need added sweetness, go for the real thing occasionally – a small amount of sugar, honey, or maple syrup – because at least your body knows how to process these.

Gut Bugs' Influence On Weight

Did you know that the type of gut bacteria we have may also affect our weight?

Our gut microbiome is mostly made up of two bacterial families, Firmicutes and Bacteroidetes. There is some evidence to support the notion that if our ratio of Firmicutes to Bacteroidetes is imbalanced, we are more likely to be overweight. That's because this delicate balance affects how well we absorb the calories from our food. If our ratio is in favour of increased Firmicutes to Bacteroidetes, we're able to extract more calories from our diet than someone who has a greater number of Bacteroidetes.

How To Shift The Balance In Your Favour

Most of us won't know what our ratio looks like – and this research is only in its early stages – however, it certainly won't do us any harm to work on increasing our Bacteroidetes, which flourish in the presence of high-fibre foods such as legumes (like beans). Firmicutes, on the other hand, do better on a sugary, processed diet!

ACTIONABLE STEPS (that you can start doing straight away)

1. Eat a variety of vegetables and fruit (mainly vegetables), aiming for up to 30 different varieties of plant foods a week – ambitious, I know! Think vegetable boxes, salads to accompany your meals, poached/baked fruit for desserts, and adding nuts and seeds to your foods.

2. Learn to love sauerkraut and kimchi, and keep them on the top shelf of your fridge – use them to garnish your meals on a regular basis.

> TIP: Keep all the foods that need eating quickly on the top shelf of your fridge so that they're visible every time you open the door. If they're hiding in a drawer or corner of the fridge, it's usually a case of out of sight, out of mind... out of mouth!

I especially like red cabbage sauerkraut because it makes all meals look so much more attractive, and don't worry – you get used to the slightly sweet taste. It's so good for you because it's literally teeming with beneficial bacteria such as lactobacillus brevis, lactobacillus plantarum, and yeasts.

My experience is that women who have added sauerkraut to their diets report better digestion all round. Start with small amounts, like a tablespoon, to avoid overwhelming your unsuspecting gut and to build up tolerance.

3. Use kefir as well as yoghurt – it contains beneficial bacteria and yeasts that are great for your gut. Add it to smoothies, put it on top of your porridge, or eat it with fruit. You can easily find kefir in most supermarkets, or you can buy the kefir grains and make your own. It's said that kefir comes from the Turkish word 'keyif', which means 'a pleasurable bliss state', and it has also been described as 'feeling well after eating'. If you're not keen on the taste, try stirring in a spoonful to your yoghurt.

4. Eat salads with avocados (yes, an avocado contains approximately 5 g of fibre, plus recall how they contain the good kind of monosaturated fat). ;)

5. Ask yourself: "Have I fed my gut bugs today?"

Introducing these foods can really encourage the growth of the more beneficial bacteria that are related to health. It can, however, take anywhere from two to four weeks to notice the benefits – so stick with it.

TROUBLESHOOTING – What happens in the gut doesn't stay in the gut!

Two of the most common complaints I see related to the gut are constipation and bloating.

Here's what can help.

TROUBLESHOOTING – Bloating

If you suffer from bloating, it's important to ensure you're not eating any foods you're intolerant to. For example, some women at midlife become intolerant to the lactose in milk and don't produce enough of the lactase enzyme to break it down. Try skipping it for a few weeks and see if it helps. Other common intolerances include wheat, corn, soya, and nuts.

Here's a list of things you can try to reduce your bloating:

Cut back on sugar – remember: it feeds the bad guys in the gut!

Chew, chew, chew, and eat your meals s l o w l y.

Try peppermint capsules – an antispasmodic that can help relieve gas, bloating, and cramps.

Add dried ginger to your food – try adding a teaspoon (per serving) to your smoothie or stir-fry. It can improve digestion and help with bloating and gas.

Avoid fruit after lunch for a while and see if this helps; it can ferment in the gut if not digested well, so try enjoying your fruit in the morning.

Avoid eating when stressed. Recall how, when you're stressed out, your body prioritises other survival mechanisms like increased heart rate and blood pressure – meanwhile, your digestion takes a back seat. This results in not enough stomach acid or digestive enzymes being secreted to break down your food – ouch!

Bloating is often connected to constipation and/or an imbalanced microbiome, where the good guys are no longer running the show – and this can result in lots of issues and poor digestive power. However, there are many reasons for bloating, and – if it's ongoing – I would recommend working with a registered nutritional therapist/dietician to uncover the underlying cause. Believe me, they're well versed on how to help you get to the bottom of it – it's one of the most common symptoms we come across.

Are You Suffering With Constipation?

Ideally, we're aiming for at least one bowel movement per day. However, you're considered to be constipated if you've gone three days without one.

It's very common to suffer from constipation during the perimenopause and menopause due to declining hormones. Recall how the digestive tract is full of oestrogen receptors, and therefore a lack of oestrogen can really slow down the muscle contraction needed for a bowel movement. Additionally, weakened pelvic floor muscles are also very common and can also result in constipation – but it's not all bad news! There is much we can do...

Try these simple tips to relieve constipation (which may also reduce your bloating):

1. Try belly breathing – just sit for 5-10 minutes and breathe slowly and deeply into the diaphragm (you can google diaphragmatic or belly breathing). This provides a gentle massaging action to the digestive tract – plus, this kind of breathing activates the parasympathetic nervous system (the calming side of the nervous system), which means your body will be more primed to let go and result in a more complete bowel movement.

2. Start your day with a large glass of water – keep it by your bedside and drink it upon waking up. Why? It will help hydrate you and may increase your urge to go. Then, keep drinking throughout the day – teas also contribute to the 1-1.5 litres of water a day you should be aiming for. Try filling a jug first thing in the morning and having it visible, such as in your office or on a countertop – it's a constant reminder to keep hydrated.

3. Get more fabulous fibre – this doesn't mean boring bran flakes (which don't, by the way, always help)! Instead, look to apples (an apple a day!), kiwis, pears, legumes, broccoli, beans, peas, nuts, and seeds (chia are great too), because they're all going to provide you with good levels of fibre. See the Feel Good About Carbs chapter and refer to the table there for more suggestions on how to gradually introduce these foods into your diet.

4. Include a tablespoon of flaxseed with your breakfast. Flaxseed is a soluble fibre, meaning it absorbs water, and this can make stools softer and therefore easier to pass. Soak the flaxseed, as in the overnight oats recipe, or add the seeds to a smoothie and let them soak for at least 20 minutes before drinking.

5. Get moving – we know that moving the body helps stimulate the intestinal tract, and therefore gets things moving in other areas too! Maybe go for a walk or do some yoga stretches before breakfast.

6. Don't rely on laxatives for too long – they can be a great relief initially, however, over time the bowel becomes too reliant on them, and bowel contraction may become weaker. Better to find dietary and lifestyle solutions that can help and that are sustainable.

7. Try a **magnesium citrate supplement** – this form of magnesium has been shown to be the most effective in

helping relieve constipation. Start with a dose of 300-400 mg daily, trying 200 mg in the morning and 200 mg before bed. Magnesium is generally well tolerated, but do check that it's OK to take alongside any medications you're already on.

8. Work on strengthening your pelvic floor muscles – this is important not just for your bowel but for your bladder too, as you may well know (achoo!). These sling-like muscles span the bottom of the pelvis and help hold up the bladder, womb, and bowel, so we really want to keep them shipshape.

To strengthen your pelvic floor muscles, sit down and squeeze them (if you have trouble knowing what to squeeze, just check out the many YouTube videos demonstrating how to do this). Imagine pulling them in and up, then hold them for 10 seconds before releasing. Repeat this 10 times daily at least.

Why not weave it into your daily habits? You could put a sticky note on your bathroom mirror to remind you, do it whilst brushing your teeth, or even when sitting at traffic lights – it's well worth the effort! There are many yoga poses – such as chair pose, happy baby, and locust pose – that can also contribute to strong pelvic floor muscles. And, if you feel you need help in this area, find a specialised pelvic health physiotherapist – they really can work wonders.

CHAPTER 14 ~ FEEL GOOD ABOUT YOUR BONES

We all want to go forward with healthy, robust bones, but we're up against it – our bone density starts declining from our thirties onwards, and drops significantly again after menopause.

Our bones are constantly building up and breaking down; they are a living tissue. Unfortunately, as our oestrogen declines, the building up bit doesn't happen as much, and therefore many postmenopausal women suffer with osteoporosis.

> It's estimated that women can lose as much as 20% of their bone mass post-menopause, and that one in two women will suffer from osteoporosis. It's never too late to start taking care of your bones.

Osteoporosis (porous bones) is a condition that weakens bones, making them brittle and fragile, therefore easier to break. It's vitally important that we do all we can to maintain our bone density in order to prevent weakened bones (bone density is simply a measurement of the amount of calcium and other minerals found in bones and is indicative of how healthy, flexible, and strong bones are).

It's a common misconception that we can just swallow a calcium pill and be done with it – unfortunately, it's much more complex than that. Let's look at what else we can do when it comes to protecting our bones.

Protein

Ensure you eat adequate protein, because 50% of bone is made from protein. This bone-protecting effect of eating protein is even better if you eat it with vegetables. Recall how you need to aim for 25-30 g with all your meals.

Vegetables

Eat lots of vegetables – evidence shows that they help increase bone density. Think a quarter to a half of your plate.

Calcium

Think of this as a building block for your bones; calcium is important for bones to maintain their hardness and durability. Aim for 1200 mg of calcium per day. As the bone cells break down and build up throughout the day, it makes more sense to have a constant supply of calcium (rather than one big dose in the morning in the form of a calcium pill).

We can only absorb approximately 500 mg at any one time – therefore, if you're taking a supplement, don't take more than 500 mg in any one dose. The evidence shows, however, that getting our calcium from food is safer and more effective. So, take a good look at the list of bone-building nutrients at the end of this chapter and build them into your diet. However, if you still feel you're not getting enough, do top up with a calcium supplement.

Vitamin D

Vitamin D is essential for bones, as it helps your body absorb calcium; without adequate Vitamin D, we cannot use calcium effectively. Whilst it's preferable to get your Vitamin D from the sun, if you live in the UK, this is impossible from October to March.

Ideally, you should be aiming for a blood level of:

50 nmol/L - 125 nmol/L of vitamin D
or
20-50 ng/ml

To attain this level, most of us need to take Vitamin D in supplement form – especially from October to March.

Based on current research, a dose of 600-1000 ius or 15 mcg - 25 mcg is adequate for most of us to reach healthy blood levels of Vitamin D. However, if you suspect you're low in Vitamin D, you may want to check your levels. There are many companies that offer a blood spot test; you can easily find these inexpensive tests online, and they can be a valuable tool in ensuring you have adequate levels.

You should also bear in mind that too high a level of Vitamin D can be detrimental to health – it's a fat-soluble vitamin and can build up in the body when taken in very high doses. However, for most of us, a test is unnecessary; we just need to be aware and take an adequate dose over the autumn and winter months.

From October until the end of March, a daily dose of 1000 units / 25 mcg is generally safe and can help you achieve an adequate blood level of Vitamin D.

Vitamin K

Vitamin K is another essential nutrient when it comes to bones, as adequate levels of Vitamin K are associated with good bone density. This is because it attaches calcium molecules to bone and prevents calcium from building up in the arteries – something we really want to avoid! Why not take a Vitamin D with added K2 supplement if you suspect you're not getting enough via your diet? (Most of us don't!)

You can find Vitamin K in leafy green vegetables, as well as natto (though this isn't as palatable for western tastes). It's also found in kimchee and sauerkraut (great condiments), some cheeses (there are good levels in Munster, Camembert, Edam, and Gouda), egg yolks, and some organ meats.

Magnesium

Magnesium is essential for many actions in the body, and it has a major role in contributing to healthy bones too. Sufficient magnesium helps with absorption and metabolism of calcium and is essential for strong bones. Low magnesium intake has been associated with osteoporosis.

If you eat a whole-foods diet, you should get adequate magnesium. However, many women feel better when taking a supplement.

Aim for 300 – 400 mg of magnesium spread throughout the day in two or three doses. Glycinate, citrate, and malate are all good forms of magnesium.

Consider Collagen

You may also like to start using collagen in your smoothie and maybe in your coffee. Collagen is the main protein found in bones; it contains the amino acids glycine, proline, and lysine, which all help build bone. Type 1 and 3 collagen are the best forms for bones. I'd recommend using it three to four times a week – like you would a food – rather than obsessively consuming it daily. The jury is still out on whether collagen, once broken down during the digestive process, can contribute to your collagen levels – but it certainly won't do you any harm in small amounts and may contribute to any missing amino acids that you need for other protein-building processes in the body. Many women that I work with tell me they feel benefits from adding it to their diets.

Practise The Right Kind Of Movement – this one is SO important!

If you can perform some strength training and weight-bearing exercises regularly – like a couple of times a week – you will promote new bone as well as increase your muscle mass/your engine/your ticket to healthy ageing!

Exercises like squats, lunges, and planks – and I know, these can be intimidating for some of us – that use your own bodyweight are great. Weightlifting is also good here, and that doesn't have to mean bench presses; what about a body pump class? Les Mills and many other companies offer online classes, and all you need is a few weights to get you started – it's basically lifting weights to music. Fitness bands are also considered a weight resistance exercise, and a lot of instructors work with these. Running, going up stairs, hiking, tennis, barre and yoga classes, and dancing are also considered to be strength training activities – basically, any exercise whereby your body is working against gravity will help you achieve more strength.

If you can, why not have a session with a personal trainer, and then ask them to show you some strength training exercises you can do on your own? Two to three sessions (of about 35 minutes) per week are considered optimal.

The Royal Osteoporosis Society recommend 50 moderate impacts daily, such as jumping, hopping, skipping, and jogging. Do take a look at their website – it's a great resource.

If walking is more your thing, then you need to know that walking alone may not help your bone mass, but what about using a weighted vest or carrying a rucksack, and making your walk a bit brisker?

Yoga – this is another activity that can contribute to great bones, because many of the poses are considered strength training. You can find many free resources online. These are two of my favourites Yoga with Adriene and Yoga with Kassandra.

HRT

Hormone replacement therapy. I include this last, but not least! We know that oestrogen has a protective effect on bones, so if you have a family history of osteoporosis – or if you feel you are in some way vulnerable – or you just want to protect your bones going forward, you may want to discuss this option with your doctor.

Avoid the following . . .

Don't Eat Less Than 1000 Calories A Day

This will not be enough to sustain you, your bones, or your muscle. Some women do this to lose weight, without realising they're compromising their bones.

Don't Let Stress Get The Better Of You

Recall how high stress = more cortisol, and this can have a detrimental effect on many things, including your bones! We really want to avoid chronically elevated cortisol, as it's what we call a catabolic hormone – meaning it breaks things down, including bones!

Don't Drink Too Much Alcohol Or Coffee/Caffeine

Alcohol can interfere with calcium and Vitamin D absorption, therefore, follow the advice here and have at least four nights off every week – as well as slowing down your consumption overall. Drink the best stuff you can afford, sip it slowly, and really enjoy it! ;)

Caffeine can increase the amount of calcium we lose in our urine, and evidence shows that drinking too much is linked with osteoporosis – you'd have to be drinking quite a lot though. It's safe to enjoy one or two cups a day, but bear in mind that most café-bought coffees include two shots, and one shot of espresso equates to approximately 63 mg of caffeine. I mention it here just in case you're a serial coffee drinker!

And, finally, smoking is detrimental to bones – in case you do smoke, now is a good time to consider giving up!

Food Sources Of Calcium
And Other Bone-building Nutrients

Food content	Quantity	Calcium/mineral
Milk	100 g	125 mg Ca
Full fat yoghurt	1 pot	207 mg Ca
Cheese, cheddar 3	0 g	240 mg Ca
Soya milk (fortified)	100 ml	120 mg Ca
Fennel	100 g	49 mg Ca
Sesame seeds	100 g	1000 mg Ca

Chia seeds	80 g		631 mg Ca
Flaxseeds	100 g		256 mg Ca
Green leafy veg	100 g		140 mg Ca
Turnip greens	1 cup		200 mg Ca
Sweet potato	1 medium potato		31 mg Mg + 542 mg K
Canned salmon	1/2 can with bones		232 mg Ca
Sardines	7 fillets		321 mg Ca
Dried figs	8		107 mg Ca
Pak choi	1 cup		74 mg Ca
Molasses	1 tbsp		172 mg Ca
Kale	2 cups		188 mg Ca
Almonds	1/4 cup	7	2 mg Ca
Oranges	1 medium		65 mg Ca
Orange juice (F)	1 cup		500 mg Ca
Soya milk	1 cup		300 mg Ca
White beans	100 g		442 mg Ca
Firm tofu (Fortified)	1/2 cup		400-861 mg Ca
Whey protein	33 g scoop		160 mg

Ca	Calcium
Mg	Magnesium
K	Vitamin K
mg	Milligram

Dried herbs: thyme, oregano, poppy seeds, rosemary, celery seed, sage, and mint contain calcium – add to foods where possible.

Prunes are a great source of Vitamin K and phenolic compounds (a powerful antioxidant). Some small studies have demonstrated that they can prevent bone loss and encourage bone formation and therefore prevent bone thinning / osteoporosis and fractures.

Aim for 5-6 prunes daily (also great for digestion and constipation!)

K2-rich foods: 180-200 mcg daily. This includes grass-fed organic animal products such as butter, eggs, dairy, meat, and organs.

FYI Vitamin K2 is predominantly found in foods that are fermented and K1, referred to above as just K is found predominantly in greens and some vegetables).

Fermented foods include **natto, sauerkraut, and kefir.**

Brie and Gouda: these aged cheeses are also an excellent source of K2.

Vitamin D levels: aiming for levels between 50-125nmol/L

Get it from the sun, oily fish, eggs, dairy, and supplement if necessary during the Autumn and Winter months.

Magnesium: 300-400 mg daily of green leafy veg, whole grains, avocado, nuts and seeds, legumes, tofu, and dark chocolate.

Calcium: 1200 mg daily.

Look at this information often until you get used to which foods are going to contribute to your bone health and maintain the strength you need for the second half of your life.

If you have osteoporosis or osteopenia, consider wearing a weighted vest to improve your bone density – however, do check with your health professional first that it's safe to do so.

Finally, if you're able to, get a DEXA scan – it's a great idea to know what your baseline is

A Dexa (Dual-energy X-ray absorptiometry) scan uses low dose x-rays to assess your bone density and assess your risk of osteoporosis.

CHAPTER 15 ~ FEEL GOOD ABOUT LEGUMES

(...AND HAVE THEM FOR LUNCH!)

Being healthy is all about having healthy habits in place, and getting into the routine of eating legumes often is a good one to work on. Legumes such as chickpeas, lentils, and beans can be so helpful in midlife, so I'd recommend having them four to five times a week. Eating them at any time is good, of course, but – being that they are so versatile – lunch is a great time to weave them into your diet.

You could also try adzuki beans, black-eyed peas, fava beans, and kidney beans.

What's So Good About Them?

Legumes can help regulate your blood sugar and improve cholesterol levels (the less desirable kind, LDL, tends to increase post-menopause) – plus, they can provide both the soluble and insoluble fibre needed to maintain a healthy gut. One cup contains one-third of the 30 g of fibre you're aiming for daily.

So, put simply, they're good for your heart and gut, they lower your risk of diabetes, they're high in protein and fibre, they're a good source of B vitamins, iron, Vitamins A and K, copper, calcium, and magnesium, and they contain phytoestrogens. What's not to like!

They're a great plant source of protein, and in midlife we're really looking to up our plant intake without compromising our protein intake. Depending on the legume, a cooked portion (1 cup/160 g) could provide you with approximately 15-25g of delicious plant protein.

They also contain lignans, a type of phytoestrogen – that is, a gentle plant-mimicking oestrogen. Remember: there is some evidence to demonstrate that higher intakes of lignans are associated with a lower risk of breast cancer and with less aggressive tumours.

> **The Mediterranean diet** focuses on fresh, seasonal foods with lots of fish, vegetables, **legumes,** and olive oil. Red meat, dairy, and processed foods take a back seat and are eaten less often. It's well established that this diet reduces the risk of all major diseases and increases longevity. And, more recently, a scientific review concluded that the Mediterranean diet is as effective as prescription drugs when it comes to helping women lose weight – which, as we know, goes on much more easily in midlife.

Changing Habits

My taste for legumes started when we moved to Spain in 1996, and it has never left me. We spent a decade living there, experiencing the Mediterranean diet first-hand. I soon observed that the Spanish made time to enjoy all their meals, and that breakfast, lunch, and dinner were all cooked from scratch. These would often be very simple meals, but they would always use fresh, nutritious ingredients.

Additionally, it struck me that the Spanish ate legumes in one form or another most lunchtimes; it's such a staple there. As I researched the connection between women and legumes, I also discovered that in the **blue zones** of the world – including Sardinia and Okinawa – they all have one dietary habit in common: that is, the regular consumption of **legumes.**

Blue Zones: What Are They?

Five Blue Zones have been identified in the world – these are geographic areas that are longevity hotspots, where you'll find a higher concentration of centenarians, and very little chronic disease. They include Okinawa (Japan), Nicoya (Costa Rica), Sardinia (Italy), Icaria (Greece), and Loma Linda (California). There are some brilliant books on the subject if you'd like to learn more.

> *The Blue Zones Kitchen* by Dan Buettner – this is a great cookbook. Dan has observed the lives of local people, up close and personal, and shared their habits along with the recipes they frequently enjoy.

So, how can we mimic this in the UK?

It's as simple as aiming for a portion a day – this simple habit can have such a positive impact on your health. A portion is often cited as half a cup of dried legumes or 1 cup of cooked – weightwise, that's anything from 120-160 g of cooked or 60-80 g of dried, they absorb a lot of water.

Start by trying at least one portion of **legumes for lunch** this week and see how you feel. And why not make legumes for lunch one of your dietary mantras? You can see the recipe section for inspiration. These recipes include chickpea salad, white bean hash, lentil and lemon soup, and Mediterranean chickpeas with tuna – all super easy to make and enjoyable to eat!

Don't, however, go too fast with legumes; if you've been eating a more processed diet, and then overnight you start eating copious amounts of chickpeas and beans, you may find you experience gut issues and become quite gassy.

Legumes can be tricky to digest – if you're not used to them – and can cause bloating initially. I'd recommend, therefore, starting with a smaller portion, or substituting rice in a 50:50 ratio if you're new to them. However, I have found that, over time, most women get used to them and are able to enjoy them regularly.

> TIP: I find that chickpeas and white beans are better when they're from jars. They tend to come from Spain or Italy and, as well as tasting superior to their tinned equivalents, people tell me they're better able to digest them. Spanish beans are cooked in softer water and retain all their flavour. You can find jars of beans in delis and some supermarkets.

Lentils, depending on the type, can be used dried and added to soups and curries. Just follow the recommended cooking time: usually 20-30 minutes.

I know that a lot of women are turned off by legumes, seeing them as boring and flavourless – but do give them a try. They can take on lots of flavour; it's just a case of finding recipes that appeal to you.

Low effort but maximum nutrition is what we're aiming for.

Here are ten ideas to get you started:

1. Use chickpeas as a base for a salad.
2. Use cannellini beans in a salad – they go well with tuna and lemon.
3. Make red lentil soups.
4. Add chickpeas to a tray of roasted vegetables.
5. Sauté garlic, then add a jar of cannellini beans and a teaspoon of horseradish and mulch.
6. Make lentil chillies.

7. Enjoy hummus on sourdough toast.
8. Whizz up cannellini beans with lemon juice, zest, and a glug of olive oil, and serve with carrot and cucumber batons.
9. Add beans to tomato sauces.
10. Roast chickpeas with a little olive oil and enjoy as a snack.

CHAPTER 16 ~ FEEL GOOD ABOUT PHYTOESTROGENS

What Are Phytoestrogens & Should We Be Including Them In Our Diet?

I've mentioned them throughout this book, so now let's have a closer look at them.

Plant oestrogens – known as **phytoestrogens** – are naturally occurring compounds that are found in certain plants. They can mimic our body's own oestrogen but in a much weaker form; they have a similar chemical structure to our own oestrogen, meaning they can sit on our oestrogen receptors. This can be useful if we have too little oestrogen – or too much. Whilst we don't want to rely on them for an oestrogen boost, the evidence certainly points to them being a helpful addition in midlife.

There are two main phytoestrogens: isoflavones, found mainly in soy products, and lignans, mostly found in seeds, legumes, whole grains, and some fruit and vegetables.

Soya has become well-established as a health food here in the UK and in the US, and you'll also find it in many processed foods! Soya, therefore, has both good and bad credentials in equal measure. Some studies conclude that its health benefits stretch to reducing the symptoms of menopause as well as decreasing the risk of osteoporosis, inflammatory conditions, and breast cancer, with other studies stating that it may disrupt our hormones and could lead to a recurrence of breast cancer.

There is no controversy when it comes to the safety of phytoestrogens in seeds, legumes, fruit, and vegetables.

There is no denying that our Asian counterparts – whose diets are rich in phytoestrogens – have a much lower incidence of breast cancer and far fewer menopausal symptoms, such as hot flushes, which makes most of us curious as to whether these plant-like oestrogens can do the same for us.

How Should We Approach These Foods?

The studies are divided, but I suspect it's a more complicated picture than just eating soya in abundance and expecting the same outcome. My approach, when replicating diets from other parts of the world, is to consider how these foods have been eaten traditionally. There are a lot of processed, genetically modified soya products out there, and you'll find soya isolate added to many foods – best avoided, in my opinion. Instead, enjoy soya in its least processed, more traditional forms.

> Asian women have certain bacteria in their guts that can convert daidzein – the isoflavone found in soya – into equol. It's the equol that has the oestrogenic properties, and it may be one of the reasons they experience fewer menopausal symptoms. It's estimated that only 30% of us in the UK have these same gut bugs, enabling us to enjoy the same benefits. Therefore, some of us will get more benefits from eating soya than others.

For most of us, eating traditionally prepared soya products three to four times a week (see list below) is most likely a good thing, and a positive step in optimising our diet. As always, listen to your body; if you start eating soya and experience digestive discomfort such as bloating, then maybe it's not for you. Or, if you decide to persevere, then just enjoy small amounts and build it into your diet slowly.

Soya is a powerhouse of nutrients; it contains calcium, B vitamins, fibre, magnesium, and potassium, and is a high-quality plant protein, making it a good meat replacement.

How Should We Approach Soya?

Stay away from highly processed soya like veggie burgers and soya cheese, and instead aim for the least processed forms of soya that have a higher nutritional value, such as:

Soya milk – organic, unsweetened.

Organic tofu (bean curd) – use in soups, curries, and stir-fries.

Tofu can soak up lots of flavours so it's a great thing to use in a curry, with spices. You can also buy tofu that is already flavoured.

Tempeh (made from whole soybeans) – this is less processed and is also fermented, hence it has the added bonus of containing beneficial bacteria. At first sight, it looks rather pale and anaemic – but marinate it and you'll find it's a great carrier of flavours.

Miso, a fermented soybean paste – this is a great base for soups; just try adding a teaspoon to any soup for added flavour. It can also be made into a hot drink or used in stir-fries, and it comes with a good dose of beneficial bacteria too.

Natto – this is another fermented soybean product, highly nutritious but not particularly appealing to an unsuspecting western palate.

Edamame beans – these beans make a great snack and are high in protein and nutrients.

The following foods contain phytoestrogens known as lignans:

Flaxseed – this is the richest dietary source of lignans, and there is some evidence to suggest that as little as 25 g a day may reduce your risk of breast cancer.

Add a tablespoon of flaxseed – which is better ground, in order to obtain its nutrients – to smoothies, porridge, or granola. Buy organic, because seeds have a large surface area, meaning they're more exposed to pesticides! And, if you have any trouble digesting them, try soaking them for 20 minutes before eating.

Legumes – like chickpeas, lentils, and white beans.

Sesame seeds – tahini is a good way of taking in these seeds, which contain lots of calcium too.

Apricots – have one or two after a meal. They're also delicious blended in porridge.

Berries – aim for a portion a day. Enjoy in a smoothie, with porridge or yoghurt, or as a dessert.

Melon – this is nice to have at the end of a meal or with breakfast.

Fennel – add grated or sliced fennel to salads, or slice a whole one into quarters and cook in the oven with olive oil.

Whole grains – such as oats, rice, barley, quinoa, and rye.

Other sources include: celery, sweet potatoes, and pomegranate seeds.

Whilst these foods may be helpful because of their phytoestrogen content, most studies show that they do seem to be favourable for most of us in general – though whether this is all down to the phytoestrogens is inconclusive. They also contain an array of other powerful nutrients, so I believe it's a good idea to weave them into your diet.

CHAPTER 17 ~ FEEL GOOD ABOUT SUPPLEMENTS

Do We Need Supplements In Midlife?

Many women turn to supplements during perimenopause and beyond, understandably looking for relief from their symptoms and wanting to ensure they cover all their nutritional needs. With so much choice out there – and with big, bold claims from manufacturers – it's easy to get drawn in and, before you know it, you have a cupboard full of supplements for every single symptom you're experiencing. However, it's much better to have a few essential, targeted supplements that will benefit you long-term.

If you do buy supplements, ensure they're from reputable manufacturers offering pharmaceutical grade products (it should say on their website), and do your research. Ask yourself: do you really need them? Also, bear in mind that it's much better to take a high-quality supplement than a cheaper, less absorbable one with lots of chemical excipients (additives). Alternatively, make yourself an appointment with a registered nutritional therapist and discuss your needs with them.

Now I'm going to share with you the top five supplements that are evidence-based, effective, and appropriate for perimenopause and menopause. These are the ones that my clients repeatedly tell me they benefit from the most.

- **Mighty Magnesium** – known as 'nature's tranquiliser', this is so helpful in midlife.

Magnesium is one of the body's most abundant minerals, and it helps with a myriad of functions in the body; it is required for more than 300 chemical reactions in the body and plays a crucial role in helping our bodies function well. Being mildly deficient in this mineral rarely results in any visible symptoms, however, a lot of us benefit enormously from taking a daily magnesium supplement.

Magnesium is helpful because . . .

It not only contributes to bone and heart heath, but it can also help regulate blood pressure and low mood (due to its influence on brain chemicals), support our adrenal glands, and help us mitigate stress, meaning our response to stress will be slightly muted. Magnesium also contributes to energy production, as well as helping our muscles to relax. It's useful in helping alleviate constipation, and many women report that it gives them a sense of calm and contributes to a good night's sleep.

It's a fairly safe mineral as long as you don't take too much. If you feel you struggle with any of the above, it's certainly worth trying a supplement to see if it helps.

Which One?

Magnesium comes in many forms. These are the ones I recommend:

Magnesium glycinate – easily absorbed and a good all-rounder.

Magnesium L-threonate – helpful if you suffer from headaches or brain fog.

Magnesium citrate – useful if you suffer from constipation.

Magnesium malate and taurate – good all-rounders.

Daily Dose

A good therapeutic dose is 300-400 mg, spread throughout the day — for example, 100/200mg with breakfast and the same with dinner or just before bed.

If you're taking medications or have any health concerns, do check with your health care provider that it's safe for you to take.

• Vitamin D

As I've said, from October to March in the UK, we don't get enough exposure to the sun to make adequate amounts of Vitamin D — hence it's essential that we supplement.

Vitamin D is vital for bone health — it helps us absorb calcium and can significantly lower our risk of osteoporosis. Vitamin D is also necessary for our immunity; low levels are associated with many diseases such as diabetes, cardiovascular disease, and some cancers. It can also help to lower our risk of contracting Covid. Remember: immunity in women can change after menopause, so we want to do all we can to support a well-regulated immune system.

It may be useful to test your Vitamin D levels; if you're low, you may need to take a higher dose for a short period of time to bring your levels back up. However, for most of us, just taking adequate amounts in winter is enough.

Vitamin D is a fat-soluble hormone, therefore if you take high doses, it can accumulate in the body — not good! You'd only do this under the guidance of a health professional if a test showed that you had very low levels.

For most of us, this is what we're aiming for:

Blood levels of 50-125 nmol/L Or 20-50 ng/ml.

From October until the end of March, a daily dose of 600 - 1000 units / 15 - 25 mcg is generally safe and can help you achieve an adequate blood level of Vitamin D.

From April onwards, expose as much skin as possible to the sun (yes, if you can, get outside in your bikini!) for 20-30 minutes – without burning, of course. The duration varies depending on your skin type, darker skins need more time in the sun to make adequate levels of vitamin D whereas fair skin types need less. Lunchtime is best. I'd always avoid the face – because my aim is to age gracefully.

If you think you may be deficient, you may want to try a finger-prick blood test, which is easy to do and inexpensive. You can easily find these tests online at:

https://www.vitamindtest.org.uk

https://medichecks.com

• **Omega-3 Fish Oils or Algae Oil**

If you're not eating oily fish, you'll most likely be deficient in these fats, and omega-3 essential fatty acids are just that: essential to health. We cannot make these long chain fatty acids hence we need to get them from our food. They are potent anti-inflammatories, which are crucial for reducing inflammation and the risk of cardiovascular disease. They may also lower our risk of arthritis, heart disease, and high blood pressure, and can be helpful for mood disorders. They may help improve our cholesterol profile too by raising our good cholesterol (HDL) and lowering triglycerides (a type of blood fat).

With so many on the market of varying quality, choose those that don't contain any heavy metals or contaminants.

And, if you're a vegan, opt for an algae oil. Cut out the middleman – e.g. the fish!

If you're eating oily fish three times a week, then you don't need these oils. If not:

Look out for oils that will give you a daily dose of Eicosapentaenoic acid and Docosahexaenoic acid, known as EPA and DHA.

Go for 1000 mg, which will typically provide you with 300 mg of EPA and DHA. The same with algae oil.

I'd recommend having some in your fridge for when you're not eating so much oily fish.

Bare Biology and **Wiley's Finest Wild Alaskan Fish Oil** are two brands I'd recommend but there are many other reputable brands.

Vivo Life Omega 3 is a pure vegan EPA and DHA supplement derived from algae.

• **B Vitamins**

During midlife, we often become deficient in B vitamins, and low B vitamin status can lead to tension, irritability, difficulty managing stress, low concentration, and anxiety.

B vitamins are a group of vitamins that work in conjunction with each other, and are usually taken as a complex. They have a far-reaching influence on our health; they're necessary for everything from energy production and hormone balance to making neurotransmitters – hence contributing to a balanced mood. They also help with the detoxification processes.

A healthy diet focusing on unadulterated, real whole foods should supply us with sufficient B vitamins. However, you may be deficient if you've been under a lot of stress, been drinking a lot of alcohol, or because you're not absorbing the vitamins efficiently.

Signs you may be low in B vitamins and might want to try a supplement include:

- Low energy
- Brain fog
- General weakness
- Low mood
- Mouth ulcers
- Mouth sores and cracks at the side of the mouth
- Headaches
- Anaemia
- Constipation
- Poor memory
- Anxiety
- You've experienced a long period of stress
- You've been drinking too much

Studies show that taking B vitamins if you're not deficient does not offer any benefits.

I'd recommend trying a B complex for 30 days and then, if you feel the benefits, continue.

Invest in a good complex with B vitamins that are in their active form – this just means you'll absorb them more efficiently.

- **Protein Powders**

If you're going to be making smoothies, you may like to try one of these powders:

Collagen

Collagen is the most abundant protein in the body, and it contributes up to 75% of our skin's extracellular matrix – in other words, most of our skin is made of it.

Collagen is not only found in our skin, but also our hair, nails, muscle, bones, ligaments, joint cartilage, and eyes – it's literally the glue that holds everything together.

I've heard one dermatologist describe collagen as being like 'ropes of protein' that, when we're young, are tightly wound, and that as we age, start to fray.

Collagen rapidly decreases in the body from our 40s onwards and, a few years after menopause, it can drop by as much as 30%. This can contribute to weaker bones and stiff joints, more wrinkles, and thinner skin. Sorry to be the bearer of bad news – but, as with all things, there is much we can do once armed with the right information.

> Don't be tempted to buy collagen face creams – they're usually a waste of time because the collagen molecule is too large to penetrate the skin and it just gets washed off!

> A recent one-year study followed 131 postmenopausal women taking 5 g (about a teaspoon) of collagen peptides daily, resulted in significantly improved bone mineral density compared to those taking a placebo.

Eating foods that stimulate collagen formation – such as greens like kale, broccoli, and spinach, as well as sweet potatoes, eggs, berries, cabbage, pumpkin seeds, garlic, orange and yellow veg, avocados, and oranges – is a step in the right direction, or you may want to try a good ethically sourced collagen powder.

If you react to fish, you can also try a **bovine** collagen powder – opt for grass-fed, which is slightly better for joints due to the type of collagen it provides.

My favourite brands include:

Bare Biology – Skinful – this is a fast-absorbing pure **marine** collagen, possibly better for the skin.

True Collagen – Ancient + Brave – grass-fed bovine collagen.

TIP: You can add two teaspoons to your smoothie or even stir it into your coffee – some brands are incredibly soluble. I add it to smoothies with a scoop of pea protein to ensure the smoothie is providing me with approximately 25 g of protein.

As with all supplements, try it and then make up your own mind. If you notice that your skin improves or that your joints feel better, then continue – if not, you may not need it, in which case don't waste your money – it's expensive!

Other Protein Powders You May Like To Try

When it comes to protein powders, opt for high-quality ones – in this case, you often get what you pay for.

Protein powders have lost their appeal for some. Nonetheless, blended into a smoothie, they can easily help you achieve your protein goals at breakfast. I've seen some fantastic results when protein powders are incorporated into diets in an attempt to provide more protein – such as more energy, fewer cravings, and weight management.

My favourite brands include:

Nuzest, Pulsin, and Motion Nutrition

Here are the different types of protein you can get:

Pea protein – a good source of high-fibre protein with branched-chain amino acids. It is helpful in muscle synthesis and is very filling.

Whey protein – a milk-based protein. This is also helpful for muscle synthesis due to its excellent profile of amino acids.

Casein protein – helpful for weight loss and muscle building.

Hemp protein – a plant-based powder that also contains healthy fats.

Rice protein – this is plant-based and digests well, but don't rely on this one too heavily; rice is a sponge when it comes to absorbing heavy metals like cadmium, which are found in some soils.

CHAPTER 18 ~ FEEL GOOD ABOUT YOURSELF

Other Ways To Look After Yourself

Having worked with many amazing women over the years, I've had the privilege of hearing their stories, struggles, and successes. Therefore, I feel I can shed some light on the areas I've observed that contribute to a more meaningful, purposeful, enjoyable, and joyful life.

This is a general and brief explanation of some areas that might provoke some thought; you can take a deeper dive into them if you wish. I hope it helps.

Find Your Tribe

"The best relationships are those you don't have to work at. If you can make a person happy just by being yourself, and they can make you feel happy just by being themselves – you've found your tribe!" – Naval Ravikant

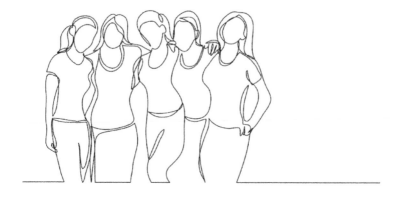

> Did you know that when bonding with friends, we produce a hormone called oxytocin, which is not only anti-ageing but also makes you feel warm and expansive!

It's important now more than ever to surround yourself with good, honest, self-aware people, as well as people that give you room to be yourself. As we age gracefully, it's so therapeutic to laugh, cry, commiserate, and celebrate life's highs and lows with those special people in your life. You should prioritise, value, and protect those relationships – they're invaluable.

Sharing your menopausal symptoms with friends is such a tonic on so many levels – you don't feel as isolated, you get access to a network of help, and it's incredibly empowering to be open and honest about your experiences.

Fortunately for us, the menopause movement – which has been happening over the last few years – means we can all start talking about how we're feeling, and thankfully, we no longer need to keep up the pretence that we're doing just fine. Phew~!

It's OK not to feel OK!

Manage Or Get Rid Of Toxic People

"Don't be reckless with other people's hearts, and don't put up with people who are reckless with yours" – Baz Luhrmann.

Other people's negativity is not your problem. If you're reading this book, you're probably over 40, meaning you have three to four decades left, so don't waste them... prioritise you!

If you feel bad or drained after spending time with certain people, then it's better to just LET THEM GO – or, at the very least, minimise the time you spend with them. Accept that relationships don't always last forever and make peace with that.

Whilst it's useful to remember that everyone is doing the best they can – and that no one is intentionally trying to screw up or frustrate you – there does come a time when enough is enough, or a break is required. Slowing down a bit gives you the opportunity to reflect upon this and do what is right for you.

Spending Time Alone

It seems that some kind of slowing-down / time alone is essential in midlife.

Time on your own can be anything from sitting outside with your coffee, reading a book, practising meditation, or just observing nature and giving yourself the space to get away from your to-do lists. This kind of practice gives you the opportunity to rest, reflect and refuel.

I call it '**me, myself time**'.

Meditation And Mindfulness

This can mean different things to different people – it could look like sitting down in a quiet place, closing your eyes, and focusing on your breath for just 10 minutes on a regular basis. It needn't be any more complicated than that.

Even doing this for 10 minutes every day has genuine benefits, such as:

Lowering stress and anxiety

Improving focus

Improving and protecting your future brain health

Why not try to find that quiet time at the beginning or end of the day, just to be on your own and follow a breathing pattern? Done regularly, it can make a positive impact; clients I've worked with report feeling calmer, less reactive in their lives, and more focused when they're able to carve out some time just for themselves. If sitting doesn't appeal and you'd rather be on the move, then build it into a walk or a cycle – or whatever does it for you. Just find a little peace and space for yourself.

Ikigai – a Japanese term for your reason for being – the thing that you live for.

Advice from a dying grandmother in Richard Linklater's film, Before *Midnight*:

"Don't be too consumed with romantic love. Friendships and work brought me the most happiness."

Purpose. A lot of us have midlife crises – or, as the French more eloquently call them, *'crise existentielle'*. This can sometimes be due to a lack of purpose or not enjoying what you do, and getting to the point where you feel it's too late to change. But it really needn't be.

Once you're back on an even keel and getting the help and guidance you need, you can refocus on what is important to you.

Some of you may already have demanding jobs and families and have your ikigai, in which case, good for you. Others may need to recalibrate. I certainly did, and that was when I chose to refocus my nutrition practice on helping women like you.

Ikigai is found by following these four principles:

1. Do what you love
2. Do what you're good at
3. Do what you can get paid for or are rewarded by
4. Do what the world needs.

Those are just the headlines, but they can provoke thought and give you an opportunity to think about what you're giving and getting from your life.

Here are some excellent books I recommend if you'd like to explore this concept further:

Ikigai: The Japanese Secret to a Long and Happy Life by Héctor García, Francesc Miralles, et al.

Ikigai: The Japanese Art of a Meaningful Life by Yukari Mitsuhashi.

Learn To Say No

This can be a tough one, but doing things that you don't want to can rob you of your time and energy, and chip away at your passion and *joie de vivre*.

Most of us have been conditioned to say yes so that we come across as helpful and likeable, whereas men generally have no problem saying no and don't waste time worrying about what people will think if they do! However, by us saying yes to everyone else, we're often saying no to ourselves.

Hence, it's important to set boundaries and take ourselves – and our time – seriously. By doing this, we're honouring and prioritising ourselves. Whilst no one wants to be difficult or unhelpful, it's essential we give ourselves the time we need to focus on what's purposeful to us.

Initially, it can feel like you're being selfish, but the reality is just the opposite. By prioritising yourself, at least some of the time, you may just find you're happier, calmer, and more joyful. Saying no can mean saying yes to being a happier person – and it's this happiness that radiates out to all those around you. Everyone deserves that!

Don't 'Mean Girl' Yourself

This is a big one. So many of us have an incredibly negative voice in our head, telling us we're not good enough, strong enough, pretty enough, slim enough, smart enough, young enough... the list goes on.

Instead of listening to all this nonsense, quieten that 'mean girl' voice and start speaking to yourself like you would to a best friend. Can you imagine telling your friends that they're too old, too weak, too fat, too lazy?! If you can, then maybe you don't have many!

Practise speaking to yourself in a kind and respectful way. And, if that voice does become critical, CHALLENGE it. Or, ask yourself: what would a good friend say to you in any given situation? It takes practice, but it can be done.

Practise Gratitude

We can get so caught up in what we don't have, what's annoying us, how much we must do, etc., that we can lose all sense of everything we have to be grateful for.

So, why not try:

1. As soon as you wake up, and before getting out of bed, start listing in your mind everything you're grateful for in your life.

You'll be surprised just how this simple act can really help put you in a positive mindset and get your day off to a good start.

2. Keep a small notebook by the side of your bed and, before you go to sleep, write down three things you've been grateful for that day.

Practising gratitude is an incredibly healthy habit to form – it is strongly associated with happiness, better mental health, and the ability to deal with adversity. It may also lead to a longer life – and a more positive one.

Good luck!

CHAPTER 19 ~ FEEL GOOD ABOUT THIS ADVICE

How To Get The Most Out Of This Advice

You may be wondering, 'How am I going to follow all this advice and put it into practice?' My aim throughout this book is to empower you with knowledge and know-how, so that you can dip in and out and gradually build these healthy habits into your life in a progressive way that works for you.

I've worked with enough people to know that simply telling them what they should be eating isn't enough to support long-term change. Instead, you need to focus on gradually instilling healthy, sustainable habits.

This is my advice to keep you interested and motivated.

Firstly, understand WHY you want to make changes – if you've got the why, you can handle the how. By this I mean go deep and ask yourself the *real* why! Write it down and put it somewhere that reminds you of your intentions daily.

Secondly, try using the feel-good four – and do it as often as possible. Just this one action is enough to have a big impact on your diet.

Thirdly, get comfortable with the timings that work for you – experiment, take your time... just find out what works, and ensure you practise a 12-hour overnight fast most days.

Then you can, gradually...

Get organised – plan your meals for the next two days, and ensure you have enough healthy and appealing food in your fridge. Remember: your environment should encourage healthy eating, so get rid of trigger foods like your favourite biscuits!

Follow the recipes that appeal to you and that you really enjoy – make them regularly until they become part of your repertoire, so you don't have to invest so much time thinking about what to eat.

Double up on the recipes – cook once, eat twice.

Follow the **legumes for lunch** rule four days a week if possible, or at least try to include them in your diet in some way.

Keep your fermented foods and healthy condiments, olives, sauerkraut, kimchi, etc. on the top shelf of the fridge so you remember to add them to your food – olives make a lovely snack and are great at staving off hunger pangs whilst you put a meal together.

Keep a drawer, box, or area of your fridge full of fresh, vital, delicious greens.

Take some magnesium and Vitamin D if you need to.

Change up your exercise or just start moving more. Do it gradually, progressing every week. If you get stuck with this, find a professional to help you – either in person or online – or find a friend in the same position as you so you can encourage each other. The more you move your body, the more you'll start to enjoy it, and the more flexible you'll be. And, what most of us forget is that by simply moving our bodies, we're gifted with more energy.

It's never too late to start. Just look at Edwina Brocklesby, now 76 years old and the country's oldest ultra-triathlete – who never used to do any exercise and took up running at 52! You don't have to be this extreme, of course; just find something that gets your heart rate up. Brisk walking, even! And don't forget: you also need to do some strength training. Invest time in finding what is an enjoyable movement for you and keep doing it!

Keep a diary – to monitor what exercise you do, how much alcohol you drink, how much yoga you do, any meditation you practise etc… just keep a diary/notebook by your bed and complete it daily. It can be so motivating to record and see your progress in black and white.

And, finally, know that you are an amazing woman with lots of experience and wisdom, and that you deserve the very best in terms of healthcare and nourishment. Don't let age, insecurity, menopausal symptoms, or hormonal imbalances stand in your way of a good, purposeful, fulfilling life. You still have so much to offer.

"Your playing small does not serve the world" – Marianne Williamson (spiritual guru to Oprah Winfrey, no less!).

Here's the quote in full:

"Our deepest fear is not that we are inadequate. Our deepest fear is that we are powerful beyond measure. It is our light, not our darkness that most frightens us. We ask ourselves, 'Who am I to be brilliant, gorgeous, talented, fabulous?' Who are you not to be? You are a child of God*. Your playing small does not serve the world. There is nothing enlightened about shrinking so that other people won't feel insecure around you. We are all meant to shine, as children do. We were born to manifest the glory of God that is within us. It's not just in some of us; it's in everyone. And as we let our own light shine, we unconsciously give other people permission to do the same. As we are liberated from our own fear, our presence automatically liberates others."

- I'm not religious. If you're not either, please replace 'God' with whatever works for you.

CHAPTER 20 ~ THE RECIPES

I've included here a selection of recipes that taste good, are great staples, and can be cooked frequently with minimum effort! They also include some of the key nutrients that are beneficial to us in midlife and beyond. I hope you enjoy them!

Many of these recipes and more are demonstrated on my Instagram account
@amandasmidlifekitchen.

Smoothies You May Like To Try

To make these smoothies, just pour the milk into a blender, followed by the other ingredients, and whizz. They all serve one, but if it's too much, save some for later.

The Purple Elixir

You will need:

- 1 cup of almond milk
- 1 cup of spinach
- 1 tbsp of almond/peanut butter (alternate between the two)
- 1 tbsp of flaxseed
- 1 cup of blueberries
- 2 scoops of pea protein (20 g)
- 1/2 an avocado

A satisfying smoothie that will keep you full until lunch. Blueberries are one of the most nutrient-rich berries around

– and they pass on their vibrancy to us. If you're planning an active morning, try adding a handful of oats and half a banana.

The Chocolate One aka The Mood Booster

You will need:

- 1 cup of milk (almond, oat, coconut, or cow)
- 1 banana (frozen works well)
- 1 tbsp of almond or peanut butter
- 1 cup of cucumber/lettuce
- 1 teaspoon of maca powder
- 1 teaspoon of cocoa powder
- A scoop or two of whey protein or pea protein (20 g)

Note: the frozen banana gives it a cool milkshake-like texture. Keep a bag of chopped banana in the freezer and you'll always have some ready to go.

The Bone Builder

- 1 cup of soya milk
- 1 tbsp of tahini
- 2 tbsp of dairy or coconut kefir
- 1 orange
- 1 tbsp of chia seeds
- 125 g of silken tofu
- 4 prunes
- A handful of greens such as spinach, chard, or kale
- A splash of vanilla extract

If you're concerned about your calcium intake, then this is the one for you. It provides you with over half your calcium needs for the day, along with adequate protein and phytoestrogens. Additionally, remember prunes have been shown to contribute to healthy bones.

The Anti-inflammatory One

You will need:

- 1 cup of soya or almond milk
- Half an avocado
- Half a medium-sized mango
- 1 tsp of powdered ginger (can be fresh)
- 1 tsp of turmeric
- A sprinkle of black pepper
- 1 tbsp of almond butter
- 20 g of pea or casein protein

The curcumin in turmeric has anti-inflammatory properties, and the piperine found in black pepper helps the body absorb it.

Why not try casein protein powder? It's a slow-digesting protein that can aid muscle growth and recovery after exercise.

Smoothies are so versatile and nutrient-dense – I hope you're inspired to try them. If you don't like the idea of protein powders, use silken tofu; it adds a creamy texture without an overpowering taste.

Amanda's Kedgeree (serves 4)

You will need:

- 1 tbsp of extra virgin olive oil
- 1 bunch of spring onions (chopped)
- 1 tsp of turmeric
- 1 tsp of ground cumin
- 1/2 tsp of ground coriander
- 1/2 tsp of ground cinnamon
- 1 large cup of rice (cooked)
- 1 packet of smoked salmon (buy wild if you can!)
- 6 soft-boiled eggs
- Fresh dill or coriander/chives

Method:

Sauté the spring onions for 5 minutes, until softened.

Add the spices and cook for a further few minutes.

Add the cooked rice and stir through.

Add the salmon (torn or cut into small pieces).

To soft boil the eggs:

Bring a pan of water to the boil.

Once boiling, gently place the eggs in using a spoon.

Boil gently for precisely 6 minutes.

Plunge the eggs into iced water.

Peel and place on top of the rice.

Finally:

Add fresh herbs – dill/chives and coriander work well.

Breakfast Or Brunch With Sweet Potatoes

I'm always looking for ways to displace bread and processed food. Here, the sweet potato doubles up as bread. This is just one idea; sweet potatoes can be used in a myriad of ways.

You will need:

- 1 medium-sized sweet potato – sliced longways
- 2/3 eggs
- 2 slices of smoked salmon/mackerel
- 1/2 an avocado
- Baked tomatoes
- Sautéed spinach
- A handful of mushrooms

Method:

Start by washing, scrubbing, and drying the potatoes – with the skins on – and then place in the oven with a splash of olive oil. Bake at 180°C for 20 minutes.

Meanwhile, place 1 or 2 tablespoons of oil in a pan and start by frying the mushrooms. Then, push them to the side of the pan and add the tomatoes. Finally, add the spinach for the last few minutes.

Serve with two eggs – either fry in a little olive oil or poach.

Take the sweet potatoes out of the oven and serve with the eggs and vegetables.

Super-Fast And Simple Lunches

Wraps

Lettuce wraps are a great replacement for sandwiches.

Use crispy romaine leaves and fill with:

Salmon or tuna, red peppers, rocket, and a splash of tamari.

Chickpeas, avocado, cherry tomatoes, celery, spring onions, and lemon juice.

Crispy aromatic duck, spring onions, cucumber, and hoisin sauce.

Smoked Mackerel Pate

You will need:

- 4 fillets of smoked mackerel
- 1 large teaspoon of horseradish
- The juice of half a lemon (to taste)
- 1 tbsp of yoghurt/crème fraîche
- Chopped fresh dill to serve

Method:

Blend all the ingredients until you get a nice chunky texture, then serve with chopped fresh dill. This is perfect to keep in a jar in the fridge, as it makes a fast lunch served with a salad and some oatcakes, or placed in a sweet jacket potato with a handful of rocket.

Sardine Pate – brilliant for bones!

You will need:

- 1 tin of sardines
- The juice of half a lemon
- 1 tsp of cumin powder
- 2 tsp of yoghurt (dairy or coconut)
- 5 cherry tomatoes
- Fresh dill to serve

Method:

Drain the sardines, then place them in a bowl and mash with a fork. Add the other ingredients and sprinkle over the dill.

Serve with a piece of sourdough or rye bread, and a handful of rocket and a few cherry tomatoes.

Note: you could replace the sardines with mackerel, if preferred. Sardines, however, are not only high in omega-3 essential fats, but also contain approx. 300 mg of calcium per tin, making them a perfect midlife food. It's nicer than it sounds!

Sweet Jackets

Method:

Take one large or two small organic jacket potatoes, then rub some olive oil and salt into their skins.

Place on a baking tray, then put in the oven at 180 °C for 25 minutes – or until a knife goes into the flesh easily.

Then, use one of the following fillings:

- Two bean chilli (see recipe).
- Mackerel or sardine pate (see recipe).
- A small tin of wild Alaskan salmon mixed with a teaspoon of yogurt, lemon juice, and a teaspoon of cumin.
- A small pot of crab served with crème fraîche, and lemon juice and zest.
- Baked beans and grated cheese.

Finally, get your greens – either grab a handful of rocket, fresh spinach, or watercress.

Tofu Salad

You will need:

- 1 heart of romaine lettuce (chopped)
- 1 organic red pepper
- 1 avocado (chopped)
- 1 small red onion (sliced)
- 1 bag of rocket or lamb's lettuce
- 1 small courgette (cut into thin slices – you could achieve this by using a vegetable peeler to achieve long, thin strips)
- 1 orange (cut to your liking)
- 200 g of tofu (Dragonfly marinated tofu is a good one)

Method:

Stir-fry the tofu in a tablespoon of olive oil and, whilst it's cooking, make the salad by placing all the ingredients in a salad bowl.

Dress the salad with the Best-Ever Salad Dressing (see below).

Place the tofu on top of the salad and enjoy! This is so tasty and a great little number for lunch. Enough for at least two serving

---

Dressings – to keep your greens interesting!

Why not keep a delicious dressing on your worktop, so that when you've steamed some broccoli or kale, you can finish it off with your favourite dressing?

Best-Ever Salad Dressing

You will need:

- 4 tbsp of olive oil
- 2 tbsp of apple cider vinegar with the mother
- 1 tsp of English mustard
- 1 tsp of honey

Place in a bottle or jar, then seal and shake.

Or:

Tahini Dressing (see recipe below)

Broccoli Salad

I love this recipe, but if you're in a rush, you can just steam some broccoli or kale and enjoy it with the tahini dressing. I return to it again and again, it's so delicious.

You will need:

- A head of broccoli
- 1 tbsp of olive oil
- 2 tbsp of pomegranate seeds
- 2 tbsp of toasted almonds

Dressing:

- 40 g of tahini
- 1/2 tsp of honey
- 2 tsp of lemon juice
- 3 tbsp of water
- 1 garlic clove (crushed)

Method:

Cut the broccoli into florets and steam for 4 minutes. Refresh in cold water, then drain and dry.

Toss the broccoli in the oil and add a little salt and pepper. Then place on a baking tray and cook in the oven at 180 °C for 30 minutes.

Crush the garlic clove and then whisk the tahini in a bowl with the lemon juice, salt, and garlic (if using). Slowly add the water half a tablespoon at a time, whisking until you have a smooth and creamy consistency.

Arrange the broccoli on a platter, drizzle the sauce over the top, and then add pomegranate seeds and toasted almonds to serve.

Legumes For Lunch

Salmon, Chickpea, And Sweet Potato Salad – (2/3 servings)

For this recipe, it's a good idea to have some poached salmon and cooked sweet potatoes already prepped – I like to have some on standby in the fridge.

You will need:

- 2 fillets of salmon (poached and flaked)
- 2 sweet potatoes (cut into wedges and baked in the oven)
- 1 small jar of chickpeas
- 1 packet of rocket
- A small bunch of spring onions (chopped)
- 1 small cucumber (chopped small)
- A handful of fresh mint (chopped)

For the dressing:

- 1 tbsp of tahini
- 2 tbsp of water
- 2 tbsp of olive oil
- A good squeeze of lemon

Method:

Start by making the dressing – simply place the tahini in a small bowl and gradually whisk in the water until you have a nice, smooth consistency. Then set it aside.

Put all the other ingredients in a salad bowl (placing the mint on last), along with the olive oil and lemon juice. Finally, drizzle over the tahini dressing.

Chickpea Salad

You will need:

- 1 jar / 400 g tin of cooked chickpeas
- 1 avocado (chopped into slices)
- 1 punnet of cherry tomatoes
- 1 small red onion (sliced)
- 1 bag of rocket
- 1 tbsp of olive oil

Optional:

- A handful of coriander or parsley
- 100 g of feta cheese

Place all the ingredients into a salad bowl and dress with the Best-Ever Salad Dressing.

2/3 servings / cook once, eat twice

White Bean Mash

You will need:

- 320 g of cooked white beans
- 1 garlic clove (crushed)
- 1 tbsp of olive oil

Method:

Start by gently heating the oil in a frying pan. Add the garlic for a few minutes and then add the beans. Push the beans around the pan for a few more minutes to incorporate all the oil and add 1 tbsp of water. Then, roughly mash the beans.

Serve with a green salad such as rocket, watercress, or spinach. And a fried egg or smoked mackerel to finish.

This is such a delicious way of cooking white beans, and it can also be used instead of mashed potatoes. Approx. 2 servings

---

Lentil And Lemon Soup

You will need:

- 2 tbsp of olive oil
- 1 large onion
- 2 garlic cloves (chopped)
- 150 g of red lentils
- 1 pint of vegetable stock
- 1 400 g tin of chopped tomatoes
- 2 tsp of tomato puree
- 2 tbsp of chopped fresh thyme
- Salt and pepper (to taste)
- 1 tbsp of lemon juice

Method:

Gently heat the oil and then cook the onion and garlic for 10 minutes, without colouring.

Add the lentils and stir, coating them well in the oil.

Add the stock and bring to the boil. Add the tinned tomatoes, tomato puree, and two-thirds of the thyme.

Bring back to the boil and then simmer gently for 15-20 minutes, stirring occasionally.

Taste for seasoning and add the remaining thyme and lemon juice. Then serve with roasted pumpkin seeds.

Note: if you want to bring the protein content up, serve with some rocket stirred into the soup or on top, a tablespoon of sauerkraut, and some sardines. This is enough for 2/3 servings.

Mediterranean-style Chickpea One Pot With Tuna And Rosemary

You will need:

- 1 jar of cooked chickpeas (drained)
- 1 onion
- 3-4 cloves of garlic
- 6 slices of chorizo
- 1 tsp of smoked paprika/turmeric
- 1 tsp of bouillon veg. stock
- 1/2 a cup of boiling water
- 1 jar of tomato sauce (we used Biona tomato and basil sauce)
- Fresh rosemary (4-5 sprigs, chopped)
- 1 jar/tin of tuna

Optional:

- Grated cheese to serve/preserved lemon

Method:

Sauté the onion and garlic for 5 minutes, then add the chorizo and paprika (and the turmeric too, if you wish).

Add the chickpeas and water, stir, and then add the tomato sauce and rosemary. Leave to simmer for 15 minutes.

Add the tuna, stir through, and then serve with a few sprigs of fresh rosemary.

Serves 2/3 - cook once, eat twice

Dinner Suggestions

The Easiest Chicken Casserole Ever

Whilst this takes just minutes to throw together, the trick is to make it in advance and then slow-cook it.

You will need:

- 8 skinless chicken thighs
- 1 clove of garlic (peeled)
- A handful of cherry tomatoes
- Fresh herbs such as basil, rosemary, and sage
- A glug of olive oil

Optional:

- Add a few potatoes or cannelloni beans

Method:

Preheat the oven to 180 °C (2 hours) or 140 °C (4 hours). It's better to cook slower!

Place the thighs in a snug-fitting casserole dish that has a lid.

Throw in the herbs, tomatoes, and garlic, and a little olive oil (add optional potatoes or beans too if using).

Place in the oven with the lid on and cook for the allotted time.

Serve with a simple green salad or some steamed tenderstem broccoli. Enough for 3/4 servings

---

Red Lentil Pasta

You will need:

- 2 tbsp of olive oil
- 1 onion (I use red but either will do – chopped)
- 1 red pepper (chopped)
- 5 garlic cloves (crushed)
- 1 tsp of paprika
- 4 sundried tomatoes (cut into strips)
- 1 tbsp of walnuts (chopped)
- 1 tbsp of tomato passata
- 1 tin of tomatoes (or a jar of tomato pasta sauce)
- 200 g of feta cheese
- A handful of black olives (chopped – optional!)
- A handful of roughly torn basil leaves
- 150 g of red lentil fusilli pasta (the twisty ones)

Method:

Gently fry the onion and garlic in olive oil until the onion is translucent and soft.

Add the paprika, sundried tomatoes, red pepper, walnuts, and olives, and stir in the tomato sauce.

Simmer for 15 minutes or longer to allow the flavours to intensify.

Meanwhile, cook the pasta – usually, simmer in a pan for 8-10 minutes.

Once cooked, drain the pasta and stir it into the tomato sauce.

Place in a bowl, crumble over the feta cheese and fresh basil, and enjoy!

Note: don't forget to serve with some greens or stir in a couple of handfuls of spinach for the last 5 minutes of cooking. Enough for 2/3 servings.

Two Bean Chilli

This is a great tasting, comforting chilli. I like to make a big pot so it keeps me going for days. Use it as a topping for sweet jacket potatoes or enjoy with a salad, or an avocado and coriander dip.

You will need:

- 1 onion (chopped)
- 4 cloves of garlic
- 1 tbsp of olive oil
- 2 tins of tomatoes
- 1 cup of chickpeas
- 1 cup of kidney beans
- 1 cup of carrots (diced)
- 1 cup of celery (diced)
- 1 cup of red pepper (chopped)
- 4 sundried tomatoes (chopped)
- 1 cup of walnuts (chopped)
- 1 fresh red chilli (chopped)
- 1 1/2 teaspoons of ground cumin
- 1 1/2 teaspoons of ground coriander

Method:

Gently fry the onions and garlic in olive oil for 5 minutes in a heavy-based pan with a lid.

Stir through the chilli, cumin, and coriander and then add the tinned tomatoes, chickpeas, kidney beans, vegetables, and walnuts.

Fill the pan with enough water until the beans are just covered.

Place the lid on the pan and cook in a slow oven for 2 hours at 160 °C.

Salmon With Garlic & Honey

You will need:

- 4 wild Alaskan salmon fillets
- Half a tsp of paprika
- 2 tbsp of butter, olive oil, or coconut oil
- 4 cloves of garlic (chopped)
- 4 tbsp of honey
- 1 tbsp of water
- 2 tsp of tamari or soya sauce
- 1 tbsp of freshly squeezed lemon
- Lemon wedges to serve

Method:

Season the salmon then set aside.

Heat the oil in a skillet-like pan under medium heat, then add the garlic and sauté for a minute, until fragrant. Then add the honey, water, and soy sauce, and combine for a few minutes.

Add the salmon to the pan, and cook each fillet (skin side down) for 3-4 minutes or until golden, spooning over the juice from time to time.

Add the lemon wedges and paprika around the salmon, baste the salmon one more time, and then transfer to a baking pan and place under a grill for a further 5-6 minutes.

Serve with steamed veg and a little rice. Serves 3/4

Tofu Stir-Fry

You will need:

- 5 spring onions (chopped)
- A 3 cm piece of ginger (finely chopped)
- 3 cloves of garlic (crushed)
- Assorted vegetables such as red peppers, carrots, broccoli, mushrooms, and fennel (chopped)
- 200 g block of tofu (chopped into square chunks)
- 1 tsp of turmeric
- 1 tbsp of coconut oil
- 2 limes

Method:

Heat the oil and start frying the spring onions for a few minutes. Then add the turmeric, ginger, and garlic, frying for another 4/5 minutes. Two servings

Add in all the other vegetables and stir-fry for 5 minutes.

Add the tofu to a wok/frying pan.

Add 1-2 tbsp of Tamari soya sauce along with the juice of 1 lime.

Serve with black or basmati rice. Approx. serves 2

Some Sides

Broccoli Salad With Tahini

You will need:

- 550 g of broccoli
- 1 tbsp of olive oil
- 40 g of tahini
- 1-2 tsp of honey
- 2 tsp of lemon juice
- 3 tbsp of water
- 1 small garlic clove (peeled and crushed)
- 2 tbsp of pomegranate seeds
- 2 tbsp of toasted almonds

Method:

Cut the broccoli into florets and steam for 4 minutes. Refresh in cold water, then drain and dry.

Toss the broccoli in the oil, along with a little salt and pepper. Then place on a baking tray and cook in the oven at 180 °C for 10-12 minutes.

Meanwhile, whisk the tahini, honey, lemon juice, garlic, and a pinch of salt, and slowly start to add water half a tbsp at a time — add just enough water to make the sauce the consistency of honey.

Arrange the broccoli on a platter, drizzle over with the sauce, and scatter over pomegranate seeds and toasted almonds to serve.

Serve with a fillet of mackerel, wild Alaskan salmon, chicken, or tofu.

Beetroot Salad – (remember great for heart and cardiovascular health)

You will need:

- 750 g of cooked beetroot
- 1 cup of natural yoghurt
- 2 tsp of cumin seeds
- 1 clove of garlic
- A handful of chopped mint/coriander

Method:

Mix and infuse the yoghurt, cumin seeds, salt and pepper, and leave for 1 hour.

Chop the beetroot into quarters, place in a beautiful bowl, and pour over the dressing,

mixing in evenly.

Sprinkle over the chopped herbs and serve.

I like to make this once a week and keep it in the fridge, to save and use throughout the week.

Sweet Potatoes – a great complex carbohydrate

You will need:

- 2 organic sweet potatoes (skins on, washed, and chopped roughly into 1.5 cm cubes)
- Sea salt and freshly ground black pepper
- 1 tsp of cumin seeds

- 1/2 tsp of fennel seeds
- Olive oil

Method:

Place the sweet potatoes into a roasting pan and add a good pinch of salt and pepper.

Add the cumin and fennel seeds and a drizzle of olive oil. Then roast in the oven for about 20-25 minutes.

Some Not-So-Sweet-But-Delicious Treats

Prune Nut Bites – makes 10-12

Every now and again we all fancy something sweet, and these nut bites are an ideal treat for midlife women as we transition through perimenopause and menopause. Enjoy them after a meal, as a mid-morning snack, or pre- or post-workout.

Prunes are fantastic for our bones. Eating just six a day has been shown to contribute to bone density.

Almonds are a good source of healthy fats, protein, and Vitamin E, making them an ideal partner for the prunes.

And, finally, the cacao powder and dark chocolate are packed full of polyphenols. These disease-fighting compounds are pro-ageing, meaning you'll age gracefully – aka slower! Dark chocolate is also a good source of iron and magnesium. Not to mention, it tastes delicious!

Method:

- 1 cup of unsalted/raw nuts (I use a combination of almonds, walnuts, and pecans)
- 1 cup of prunes (pips removed)
- 3/4 of a cup of peanut or almond butter
- 1 tsp of vanilla extract
- 1 tbsp of cocoa (chocolate) powder
- 100 g of dark chocolate (melted)
- Edible petals – optional

Method:

Start by blitzing the nuts in the blender, then add all the other ingredients until well combined. Next, roll into small balls.

Melt the dark chocolate in a bowl over a pan of hot water, known as a 'bain-marie'.

Place the balls on a baking sheet and drizzle over the melted chocolate with a small spoon.

If using edible flowers, sprinkle these over now – whilst the chocolate is still melted.

Refrigerate for 30 minutes or until the chocolate has set.

Note: these freeze well and will keep in a sealed container for 4-5 days.

Cashew Nut Pudding

Cashews are low in sugar and rich in fibre, healthy fats, and protein – as well as providing us with healthy minerals such as magnesium.

Try it – you won't be disappointed!

You will need:

- 1 large handful of cashew nuts
- Half a cup of milk such as coconut milk, almond milk, or cow's milk
- 1 heaped tsp of cocoa powder
- 1/2 tsp of vanilla essence or paste

Method:

Place all the ingredients into a blender and whizz until completely blended. Adjust milk to desired consistency and then pour the mixture into ramekins, chilling for 30 minutes.

So deliciously simple!

Whole Apple Crumble – serves 1

You will need:

- 1 apple (this is one serving, but double up and have one for later)
- 1 tsp of jam
- 1 tsp of butter
- 1 tsp of walnuts
- 1 tsp of pumpkin seeds

Method:

Start by coring the apple, but don't go all the way through – keep it whole.

Place the jam inside the apple, along with the butter, and use a little for the base of the apple to keep it in place on a baking tray.

Once the apple is on the baking tray, place it in the oven for 35 minutes at 170 °C.

Top with chopped walnuts and pumpkin seeds (you could toast these first in a frying pan), then serve with yoghurt or a little cream.

This tastes like apple crumble, but without any of the sugar. The pectin in cooked apples is very gut-friendly.

Chia Pudding

You will need:

- 2 tbsp of chia seeds
- 100 ml of almond or coconut milk
- 1 tbsp of plain unsweetened coconut yoghurt
- 1 tsp of powdered cinnamon or cardamon

Method:

Place in a bowl and whisk all ingredients together.

Pour into a glass cup or ramekin and place in the fridge for a few hours (or overnight).

Then, serve with one of the following toppings.

Topping Ideas:

- Chopped mango and coconut shavings
- Fresh berries and grated dark chocolate
- Grated dark chocolate and a dessertspoon of chopped walnuts
- 1/2 a cup of pomegranate seeds, blueberries, or raspberries.

Orange Cake

A delicious moist cake which is fabulous served warm or cold and accompanied with a dollop of yoghurt. This recipe uses the whole orange, including the peel, which is full of some really good plant compounds – plus, you'll be maxing out on the fibre and Vitamin C. Make sure you buy organic as you don't want to be subjected to pesticides. The olive oil also crams in some healthy anti-inflammatory fats.

You will need:

- 2 oranges left whole (organic/non-waxed)
- 250 g / 9 oz of ground almonds
- The zest of 1 lemon
- 4 free-range eggs
- 3 tbsp of olive oil
- 60 g / 2 oz of honey or coconut sugar
- 1/2 tsp of sea salt
- 1 tbsp of bicarbonate of soda

Method:

Wash the oranges and then gently boil them for 1 and a half hours, or until soft.

Place the whole oranges (peel and all) in a food processor and blend until smooth.

Add the lemon zest, eggs, honey or coconut sugar, oil, ground almonds, salt, and baking powder until thoroughly mixed.

Pour the batter into a greased 9-inch round cake tin.

Bake in the oven at 180 °C for 45-50 minutes, until a knife comes out clean.

Cool in the tin before taking out.

ABOUT THE AUTHOR

With over a decade of experience, Amanda Ryder (BSc) is a registered nutritional therapist who is committed to helping women as they approach menopause. Amanda runs her own practice in Cambridge, helping women from all walks of life to navigate menopause, improve their health and energy, and embrace their midlife.